1988

CARING FOR YOUR OWN

Nursing the Ill at Home

Darla J. Neidrick, R.N.

WILEY

John Wiley & Sons, Inc.

New York • Chichester • Brisbane • Toronto • Singapore

Publisher: Stephen Kippur
Editor: David Sobel
Managing Editor: Andrew Hoffer
Assistant Managing Editor: Corinne McCormick
Editing, Design, and Production: Publications Development Co.
Illustrator: Brian Pendley

Library of Congress Cataloging-in-Publication Data

Neidrick, Darla, 1947–
    Caring for your own: nursing the ill at home / Darla Neidrick.
    Bibliography: p. 233
    ISBN 0-471-63702-5
    1. Geriatric nursing.   2. Aged—Home care.   I. Title.
RC954.N35   1988
649.8—dc19   87-33250
                                                                    CIP

Printed in the United States of America

88 89 10 9 8 7 6 5 4 3 2 1

PREFACE

Caring for Your Own: Nursing the Ill at Home is written for those special persons who choose to take an ill family member into their home for care. This book is especially for those families who will be giving nursing care, even though they have little or no medical background. Medical advances are appearing at a faster and faster pace. Hospital stays are being shortened, which means that the patient and family have more responsibility for medical and personal care. More than ever, both patient and family need to have basic medical knowledge and general nursing skills in order to administer care properly.

The book begins with the decision of whether or not a family should take an ill loved one home for care. The many aspects of care in the home are discussed including setting up the sickroom and obtaining special equipment. Also included are procedures for physically caring for the ill at home, such as bathing the patient, checking the temperature and pulse, planning good nutrition and special diets, caring for the skin, planning activities and exercise, dealing with bowel and bladder problems, and preparing and giving medications.

Almost daily in my work as a visiting home health nurse I see patients and their caregivers make mistakes, some serious and others not so serious, simply because they do not know what to do. Caregivers need access to much basic knowledge to properly perform their role. Confidence and good patient care come with basic medical knowledge and basic nursing skills. In order to assist both patient and caregiver, I include some general signs and symptoms that should be reported to the physician and how to properly describe those signs and symptoms.

The growing elderly population has special problems of which the younger population is not aware. These problems are discussed from both an emotional and physical standpoint so that the person administering care has better insight as to why an elderly loved one behaves or feels a particular way.

Caring for Your Own: Nursing the Ill at Home deals with the basic nursing care that will benefit any adult suffering with a long-term illness or a debilitating condition requiring care in the home.

The decision to take an ill family member into your home is not an easy one. Just as the patient has special problems, so does the caregiver as well as the caregiving family. The physical and emotional problems of caregivers cannot be ignored. I discuss general problems of caregivers and offer hints on coping with an ill family member in the home in order to ease the burden of the caregiving family. My aim is not only to promote physical and emotional well-being for the patient, but to promote physical and emotional well-being for the caregiving family so that all members of the family, young or old, sick or well, live together happily and harmoniously.

Although it may be difficult for you to think of your ill loved one as a "patient," the term is used in this book for clarity to describe the wide range of individuals who receive care.

Where we have used male or female personal pronouns, please remember that the caregiver may be a husband, a wife, sister, or friend. Neither gender nor relationship are specified in the term "caregiver."

This book is a guide and is not intended for diagnostic or treatment purposes. *Always consult and follow the advice of your physician.*

Darla J. Neidrick, R.N.

ACKNOWLEDGMENTS

My special thanks and deep appreciation are expressed to Linda Atkins, a caregiver; Deborah Beers, R.N.; Bernie Clark, R.D.; Sally Evans, R.N.; Lynn Gilham, B.S., M.Ed.; James McLarren, R.P.T.; George O'Neil, R.P.; Mary Whitehead, R.N.; Merry Jo VanCleve and the Philipsburg Library staff, Philipsburg, Pa.; Life Support Products, Houtzdale, Pa.; American Heart Association; Alberto Culver Company; Carnation Healthcare; C.B. Fleet Company, Inc.; E.I. duPont de Nemours & Company; American Lung Association; National Association for Hearing and Speech Action; National Association for Visually Handicapped; Procter & Gamble Company; Ross Laboratories; and my patients and their families.

CONTENTS

INTRODUCTION: THE DECISION

▶ YOU, YOUR FAMILY, AND YOUR PATIENT

The problem of what to do with an ill family member—be it a mother, father, sister, brother, aunt, or uncle—who is no longer able to properly care for himself is one that many families are facing. Besides considering the rising costs of nursing home facilities, you may feel your family member is not really ill enough to be confined to an institution or that he or she would be unhappy living there.

There are many factors to consider in deciding whether to bring an ill family member into your home. All persons, regardless of age and mental and physical condition, deserve kindness, respect, and the best care that can be given. Most importantly, they deserve love. Both you and your family should be willing to give loving care to the person you take into your home, not because you feel obligated, but because you genuinely care about that person's well-being. That person, even if mentally confused, will sense whether your love is genuine.

Consider your own feelings very carefully regarding this delicate matter. Perhaps you are a middle-aged housewife who has finally reached the point in life when your children are grown or near grown and no longer need your constant support. You have finally reached that era when you are able to devote some time strictly to yourself. You may resent the invasion of an ill person at this time. Perhaps you and your spouse have finally reached that time when you can devote more time to each other. The addition of an ill person could destroy that special time. Remember, too, that this person is ill, and it is human nature to let the worst of one's personality slip out during an illness.

Consider your own health and the health of other members of your immediate family. You will have to be in the best possible physical health in order to administer good care to an ill person in your home. The patient who is weak and confined to bed will need to be turned and have frequent position changes. You need to be physically strong and have plenty of endurance to help lift a patient out of bed.

The mentally confused person might not seem like much of a physical burden, yet tending to this patient can be even more physically and emotionally draining. The confused person's behavior may resemble that of a two-year-old, asking the same questions over and over and repeating the same stories time after time. To deal with this person daily demands that you be emotionally fit and in good control of your own feelings. You must have understanding, maturity, compassion, and an even temperament. If you feel you fly off the handle easily, you should not consider caring for a senile person. If you or another member of your immediate family is physically or emotionally ill, you cannot consider caring for an ill person in your home.

Consider the other members of your family before you consent to take an ill person into your home. Even if a loving relationship with your spouse has existed for many years, your spouse may resent and actually be jealous of the time and attention you must now devote to your patient. These feelings might not be apparent at first, and more than likely your spouse would deny or would not even recognize them, but eventually your marriage may suffer. Teenagers in your home may also have difficulty adjusting to a new member, and the same feelings of anger, resentment, and jealousy may occur. Have frank, honest talks with all family members before you make any decision about taking an ill person into your home.

For a spouse to insist upon bringing an ill parent to reside in the home against a husband's or wife's wishes will only cause a great strain on the marriage. If you have not gotten along with your father-in-law or mother-in-law for the last 30 years, do not think that because you welcome him or her into your home, the situation will improve. More than likely your relationship will deteriorate.

If the ill person needs constant supervision, you could become a 24-hour-a-day babysitter. You will need the support of your spouse and all other members of your immediate family. Make it known that you expect them to assist with caring for your patient whenever possible. Stress that this commitment is not your sole responsibility, but as a family you are all responsible for your patient's care and well-being. If your family members express the same feelings of fondness and love that you feel for this person, they will be willing to assist with caregiving. For even more assistance, consider employing someone outside your home, such as a nurse's aide, either on an occasional or routine basis (see Chapter 1).

Problems could develop between you and your patient regarding roles in the household. Perhaps you are a daughter thinking of bringing your mother to live with you, but your mother has always been domineering toward you. Your mother may not be able to accept the fact that she is no longer in control and that you would be in control of your household. She may continue to try to dominate and perhaps take over your own home. The same problem can arise between a son and his father.

There are situations when one particular daughter or son is selected by other sisters and brothers as being "the logical choice to take mother or father into your home." Do not allow other family members to persuade you to make a decision because you are the most likely candidate to care for an ill relative. Too often a family member is made to feel guilty and is pushed into a decision because sister Anne has a full-time job or brother Jim's home is too small.

The decision to take an ill person into your own family should be made only by you and members of the immediate family who will be involved with the care. Only you can decide if you and your family are prepared to make the necessary changes in lifestyle and give up some of your independence.

You may also have reservations about actually being capable of giving the necessary care the patient needs. If your loved one has a complex illness, care may be better provided in a nursing home setting. Naturally you will have some fears about caring for an ill person in your own home, but you should feel you are capable of learning the necessary skills to administer proper care. Depending upon the actual physical and mental condition of your patient, these skills, which include practicing good skin care, providing nutritious meals, and assisting with medications, are not difficult to learn. With common sense and practice, you will be surprised how quickly you and other family members are giving good care to your patient.

Not only will this be a drastic change in lifestyle for you, but it will also be a drastic change for your patient. The desires of the patient in question should not go unheeded. A strong-willed individual who has vowed never to be a burden to his family may feel guilty about coming to your home. The patient may feel more comfortable and more independent going to a nursing home to live.

You should be familiar with your particular patient's personality and quirks. With aging, the adjustment to change is more difficult. Consider the feelings of the patient regarding this matter. Try to put yourself in his place. An independent, 80-year-old person who has spent the last 50 years living at the same home will be reluctant to give up this independence. This sounds like a depressing situation, and indeed, the elderly are prone to depression. You may have to deal with mood swings and perhaps personality changes that have occurred due to illness. (More about depression is discussed in Chapter 10.)

An elderly person is also usually very set in his ways and routines. Maybe he always arose at 4 A.M. and had breakfast by 4:30 A.M. Perhaps he is willing and able to adjust to your routine of arising at 6:30 A.M. or perhaps he is not. You, your family, and your patient will all need to adjust and compromise, but this will be more difficult for the elderly patient, who will feel threatened by the drastic changes in his life. In addition, the patient may no longer feel in control of his own life. He may become extremely stubborn or selfish. Frustration and anger are common, although this does not mean that he is angry at you. He is angry and frustrated over his illness and the many changes in his life. Avoid judging him too harshly; ill health and changing homes have caused a great upheaval in his life.

Other difficult situations may arise. You may have to deal with a patient who is depressed and cries easily or one who attempts to run away several times a day. At times, the patient may be too dependent upon you and your family. He may be or become senile and could have hallucinations. Arguments may erupt. Suicide is a fairly common problem among the elderly.

Talk with other families who have taken an ill person into their homes. Ask about their problems and how they coped. Although their situations are not the same as yours, and every family and patient will have problems that are unique to them, you will discover some of the problems that can arise.

On the positive side, the lives of families and patients have been greatly enriched because they have chosen new lifestyles and living arrangements. Many families composed of a grandparent, husband and wife, and teenage children live compatibly together in an arrangement in which each age group draws support from the other and gives support in return. Their lives are drawn much closer together. Teenagers especially discover and learn to love and admire a grandparent whom they have known only casually until now.

Most caregivers find a deep sense of fulfillment in caring for an ill family member at home. The care you give will be of a more personal and loving nature than your patient could receive in a nursing home setting.

As the caregiver, sometimes you will be angry and frustrated. At other times, you might actually feel some of the pain your ill patient is experiencing and suffer along with him. For most, however, the love between the patient and family flourishes and grows. Their bonds are strong and enduring.

It is possible to invite an ill person into your home and administer the best of physical care, yet completely forget the emotional needs of that person. Although the patient lives in the same home, he may spend his time shut up and isolated in his room and never be really included as a family member. Mental neglect is the cruelest treatment of all.

Weigh all the pros and cons carefully before you make a decision to take an ill person into your home. This will be one of the most difficult decisions you and your family ever have to make. To help with this decision, questionnaires are included for the primary caregiver, other family members, and the patient. Each family member should answer his questionnaire honestly and anonymously. Participation by the ill person will, of course, depend on that person's condition. Then plan a family meeting to discuss the responses and help guide you with your decision.

▶ Questionnaires

Questionnaire for the Primary Caregiver

1. Do you genuinely care for and love this ill family member?
2. Has your past relationship with this person been good?
3. Do you enjoy being with older and/or ill persons?
4. Are you willing to give your patient the best physical and emotional care possible?
5. Do you have time to devote to your patient's care and well-being?
6. Would you accept the time you must spend with your patient without resentment?
7. Are you physically and emotionally capable of caring for your patient?
8. Are you capable of learning the skills necessary to care for your patient properly?
9. Are you kind and considerate of others?
10. Are you patient, tolerant, and understanding of others?
11. Are you able to compromise and adjust easily?
12. Are you willing to comply with ground rules regarding schedules, mealtimes, quiet times, and so forth?
13. Would you accept the physical changes and alterations to your home?
14. If your patient has a limited income, do you have the financial means to care for him adequately?
15. Your patient's condition could deteriorate. Are you willing to face the possibility that he might die while in your care and perhaps in your home?
16. Will you include your patient as a family member?
17. Have you considered the wishes of your other family members?
18. Are other family members willing to participate in your patient's care?
19. Do you feel obligated to take this ill person into your home?
20. Would you resent the time you must give up spending with other family members?

21. Are you being forced into this decision?
22. Do you lose your temper easily?
23. Do you expect a monetary reward for caring for your patient?
24. Would you resent the interruption of your own daily (and sometimes nightly) schedule?
25. Do you tease or make fun of senile persons?

If you answered questions 1 through 18 "yes" and 19 through 25 "no," this may help you with your decision of taking an ill person into your home.

As the person primarily responsible for the patient's care, you must feel comfortable with your decision to take this person into your home. Your decision must be based on love and concern for the ill person. You must have an even temperament and be willing to spend as much time as necessary with your patient daily. Do not expect to be paid for your services; consider them acts of love.

Questionnaire for Other Family Members (Secondary Caregivers)

1. Do you genuinely love and care about the well-being of this ill person?
2. Has your past relationship with this person been good?
3. Do you enjoy being with older and/or ill persons?
4. On a daily basis, are you willing to devote some of your time to your patient?
5. Are you willing to give the best physical and emotional care possible?
6. Would you accept the time you must devote to your patient without resentment?
7. Would you accept the time your spouse/parent devotes to your patient without resentment?
8. Are you physically and emotionally capable of caring for your patient?
9. Are you capable of learning the skills necessary to care for your patient properly?
10. Are you patient, tolerant, and understanding of others?
11. Are you able to compromise and adjust easily?

12. Are you willing to comply with ground rules regarding schedules, mealtimes, quiet times, and so forth?

13. Would you accept the physical changes and alterations to your home?

14. Are you willing to face the possibility that your patient might die and perhaps in your home?

15. Will you include your patient as a family member?

16. Have you considered the wishes of your other family members?

17. Do you feel obligated to take this ill person into your home?

18. Are you being forced into this decision?

19. Do you lose your temper easily?

20. Would you resent the interruption of your own daily (and sometimes nightly) schedule?

21. Do you tease and make fun of senile persons?

22. Would you no longer feel free to invite friends and/or business associates to your home?

23. Would you resent a change in your lifestyle?

If you answered 1 through 16 "yes" and 17 through 23 "no," this may help you with your decision of taking an ill person into your home.

All family members should feel comfortable with the decision of taking an ill person into their home. They should be willing to participate in care without resentment and be understanding of the time and energy which will be directed to the ill person. All family members must be kind, tolerant, and willing to compromise. This decision must be based on love and a genuine willingness to help the patient. Although there will be some physical changes in the home, these changes, whether minor or major, should not affect any family member's concept of his home.

Questionnaire for Your Patient

1. Do you love and care for this family?

2. Has your past relationship with this family been good?

3. Do you enjoy being with younger persons?

4. Do you feel this family is physically and emotionally capable of caring for you adequately?
5. Do you feel this family is capable of learning the necessary skills to care for you properly?
6. Are you willing to adjust and compromise as needed?
7. Are you tolerant and understanding of others?
8. Are you kind and considerate of others?
9. Will this family include you as a family member?
10. Are you willing to comply with ground rules regarding schedules, mealtimes, quiet times, and so forth?
11. Are you willing to pay your fair share of household expenses?
12. Have you considered the wishes of all family members?
13. Do you feel obligated to live with this family?
14. Do you lose your temper easily?
15. Would you feel yourself a burden to this family?
16. Would you feel more comfortable living in a nursing home or boarding home environment?

If you answered 1 through 12 "yes" and 13 through 16 "no," this may help you with your decision of establishing new living arrangements with this family.

Your decision should be based on your love for the caregiving family and their love for you. You must be willing to make adjustments and become "one of the family." You should not feel you are an imposition on the family.

CHAPTER 1

HELP FOR THE CAREGIVER

▶ ESTABLISHING A TIME PERIOD

After discussions with your family and the ill person have concluded that no member involved is against new living arrangements, decide upon a specified trial period. Your arrangements need not be permanent. For example, set a date six months from now to reevaluate your living arrangements and determine if it is in the best interest of everyone involved to continue the arrangements or make changes. Agree upon a temporary arrangement for a specified amount of time with the patient.

Everyone has heard of situations such as the one in which an elderly grandmother moves in with her daughter's family just long enough to recuperate from surgery. However, after the grandmother is well, she stays on. Years later she is still residing with her daughter's family. You have probably also heard the example of the terminally ill patient who was given six months to live and instead lived six years.

Be sure your patient understands that this is a temporary arrangement—a trial period for *everyone* involved.

▶ FINANCIAL AND LEGAL MATTERS

Ground rules are needed just as for every family sharing a home. For some families, these rules are unstated, but all members know the rules. These rules need to be made explicit for the person joining the family unit. Since having another person living with you will undoubtedly strain your budget, the patient should expect to share household expenses. A specific amount of money should be agreed upon. If you plan to hire outside employees such as a nurse's aide to assist from time to time, money will need to be set aside for this expense. Consider whether outside help to assist with household chores will now be needed, too.

This is an ideal time to discuss any financial or legal problems with your family attorney. Because you have decided the living arrangements will be on a temporary basis, do not make any drastic decisions such as the selling of your patient's former home. However, discuss legal matters such as attaining power of attorney, wills, and burial arrangements.

▶ COPING WITH THE ELDERLY PATIENT

Coping with the elderly patient who is now a member of your household could be one of the most frustrating experiences of your life; on the other hand, it could be one of the most gratifying. The results will depend upon your patient, yourself, and your family. Some elderly patients fit in well with their new family, while others are a constant source of worry and frustration. As the caregiver, you will discover that some days will be good and others will be less than perfect.

If the elderly person is in fair health and only residing with you while recovering from surgery, you will see a gradual improvement in his condition, and it will be rewarding to see the patient become well again. But many persons suffer from chronic, debilitating diseases. Chronic conditions slowly take their toll and it is not pleasant to watch an active, intelligent person whom you love suffer with a chronic illness such as Alzheimer's disease. They lose control of bowel and bladder function, and mental deterioration makes them incapable of putting a few words together to complete a sentence. Just as this type of condition will be devastating to your patient, it will be every bit as devastating to you and your family.

It is difficult to cope with such an illness and live with this person on a daily basis. There will be days when you are frustrated and depressed, with only the prospect of the days and weeks to come being filled with yet more frustration and depression. You may feel some of the same feelings your patient is feeling, such as hopelessness, guilt, and despair. Certainly there will be times when you may say to your patient, "I know how very sick you are," and you can sympathize with him; however, for you to constantly talk about your patient's crippling illness every time you walk into the sickroom would only help to destroy his morale. To say instead, "I know you are very sick today, but there have been bad days before, and there will be good days just ahead," would help the patient feel that all is not hopeless. Even the terminally ill patient needs to have a sense of hope.

▶ THE DEPRESSED CAREGIVER

Dealing with a patient who is constantly depressed and moody can lead the caregiver to feelings of depression and moodiness. First, you will need to deal with your patient's depression. Consult your family physician and seek the help of mental health counseling if necessary. Then confront your own feelings. Your depression could be caused by your patient and by your situation. You could feel lonely, isolated, and bored. Do not be afraid to admit and discuss your feelings. Talk with your family, physician, and clergyman. If there are support groups in your area, join them. There are many Alzheimer's support groups, and anyone dealing with a mentally confused patient would benefit from attending their meetings. There are also multiple sclerosis support groups, sight loss groups, stroke support groups, and so forth. Consult the local county health association for groups in your area. If you know of other families in the area who have an ill member residing with them, consider forming your own support group. You will be amazed how easily you can discuss your problems with others coping with the same situation. You will find the solution to problems that have been troubling you, and in return you will have the solution to help others with a problem of home care.

If you often find yourself crying and depressed, eating poorly and losing weight, or uncaring about your own appearance, these signs and symptoms should be brought to the attention of your physician. Just as you would seek help for your mentally depressed patient, you must also seek mental health counseling for yourself.

▶ THE FRUSTRATED AND ANGRY CAREGIVER

There will be times when you become angry and frustrated. For example, your patient has no control of urine and bowel function. You have just finished bathing him, giving special attention to the genital and rectal areas. The patient is settled into the recliner when he tells you he has to go to the bathroom. You help the patient from the recliner, take him to the bathroom, and then discover he has been unable to wait. You feel angry and frustrated. You want to verbally lash out at your patient. You may even feel that he has done this just to anger you.

At times like this, you must gather all your emotional strength to remain calm. The old remedy of slowly counting to ten when angry will help. Above all, stop and think before saying or doing anything. No one intentionally soils himself (or spills food, or loses pills in the bedcovers). Yes, you will have to start all over again but be understanding and calm. Always treat your patient with love and respect.

If incidents such as these are common, and you find yourself becoming angry many times throughout the day, you will have to admit to yourself that you need the assistance of others to help care for your patient. This assistance can come from within your family, or you can employ outside help to relieve you for a specified number of hours a day.

▶ COPING WITH THE DEMANDING PATIENT

The demanding patient may prove to be both physically and emotionally draining. Perhaps every time you leave the patient's room you are called to return to perform a simple task, such as rearranging the pillows or handing him a glass of water. Consider your patient's motives for such action. The person could actually be saying, "I'm lonely," or "I'm afraid to be left alone." Of course, you will want to anticipate any needs as much as possible. Make sure the patient is comfortable before you leave the room, and have all items that could be needed within easy reach. You should also encourage your patient to be as independent as possible.

Tell your patient where you will be in your home and when you will be returning to his room. Perhaps he could sit in the living room while you are in that room. If your efforts are futile and your patient remains demanding, hire a companion for your patient for at least a few hours each day. Possibly there are volunteer groups in your area who can help with this. There may be a teenager in the neighborhood who would tend to your patient for a few hours each evening or through the dinner hours when your schedule is hectic.

Consider Mrs. A. She suffered from arthritis and chronic lung disease for many years and had become increasingly weak and demanding. Her family hired a companion from 9 A.M. to 12 P.M. each weekday. They found that having a companion for only three hours a day was a great relief in coping with their demanding patient. The entire family's attitude changed after the companion was hired.

Humor is a valuable tool for both you and your patient. Of course, you would not want to laugh at the patient; laugh with him. Your own sense of humor may help you through many difficult situations in which you would have otherwise reacted with anger, frustration, or hostility.

A confused patient, Mrs. C., seemed to think she was living in a hotel instead of her home. She constantly got her family's attention by calling out, "The lady in room two would like two pancakes for breakfast." If the family did not immediately respond, she would call out, "The lady in room two would like three pancakes for breakfast." The pancake order increased each time she called out. Much to this family's relief, they were able to see the humor in this request, and they often jokingly asked each other and Mrs. C. how many pancakes had been ordered that morning.

Sleepless Nights for the Caregiver

Certainly you cannot perform at your best after being awakened several times each night to care for your patient. Needless to say, this will also put a great strain on your sex life, and in turn your marriage will suffer. Perhaps other family members will take over your patient's morning care on weekends, so you can sleep an extra hour or two.

Some families have solved this problem by hiring a companion to "sleep in" three or four nights a week.

Other Feelings of the Caregiver

At times you may feel sorrow and pity for your patient. Sometimes you will feel anxious, frightened, and worried about his physical health. You may feel abandoned, isolated, and tied down. These are all normal emotions that you will feel from time to time. It is only natural to feel sorry for your patient occasionally. After all, your loved one is ill, and sometimes all your best efforts do not seem to help him feel better.

If there are times when you are particularly worried about your patient's actual physical or mental condition, help is usually just as far away as your telephone. Call your physician if you think there has been a change in your patient's condition. If you cannot reach your physician, help is available 24 hours a day at the local hospital emergency room.

Another common complaint of the caregiver is being constantly fatigued and worn out. If this is a problem, perhaps you are trying to do too much. Perhaps too much burden and responsibility has been placed on you. Also, caregiver fatigue could be caused by the simple boredom of performing the same tasks over and over for a long period of time.

To help with patient care, housework, and cooking meals, pace yourself and work in an organized fashion. For example, do not start four tasks, racing back and forth among them. Work on one task at a time. When it is completed, rest for as long as you feel necessary to revive your energy and congratulate yourself for completing that task instead of thinking of ten more to do. If you are a homemaker who had once prided herself on a spotless home, you may now find that it cannot be kept as immaculate as it once was. Avoid fretting over your home. You have new priorities now, and your patient and family are at the head of the list.

Delegate chores to other family members. Remember to praise them for their assistance; a "please" and "thank you" are always appreciated. Hire someone to help with housework and/or yard work. At least get help for the heavy housework and housecleaning. If your duties also include cooking, try to conserve energy by preparing large amounts when you have time and freezing the extra for those days when you are unusually busy with your patient. Instead of making one casserole, for example, prepare two while you have all the ingredients out. Perhaps your spouse or a teenager in your home will enjoy preparing dinner one or two evenings a week.

Fast-food takeouts are fine for an occasional meal, but when ordering from a fast-food restaurant examine the nutritional content. Consider the salt, fat, and cholesterol contents. The meal should contain a balanced diet from the four basic food groups. Perhaps there is a home-style restaurant in the area that would prepare meals for you to take out.

TV dinners are easy to prepare, but again you must examine the nutritional value and salt and fat content. You can also use a microwave oven for faster preparation of meals. Save leftovers and make your own TV dinners to reheat in the microwave.

When days are hectic, make your workload as light as possible. Use all the labor-saving devices available (automatic clothes washers and dryers, dishwashers, and microwave ovens). If your spouse insists on ironed shirts, send them to a laundry.

You might find an occasional cobweb in a corner now, and your meals might not have that "slaved over the stove for hours" touch they once had, but look at what you do have. You have a family and a patient you love, and they in turn love you. Love, happiness, and harmony are important. Ten years from now you will have long forgotten that cobweb in the corner, but you will always remember your patient's smile when you took the time to soothe that aching back with a back rub.

Questionnaire for the Caregiver

As a gauge of your own emotional well-being while caring for your patient, ask yourself the following questions.

1. Are you crying or feeling blue a good deal of the time?
2. Are you often frustrated or angry? Are you taking out your anger or frustration on yourself, your family, or your patient?
3. Are you losing your temper too often?
4. Do you often pity yourself and your situation?
5. Are you resorting to the use of pills or alcohol to help get through the day?
6. Is your appetite poor, and are you losing weight?

7. Are your attire and appearance sloppy and uncaring?
8. Are you neglecting yourself or your family?
9. Are you constantly tired?
10. Are you neglecting your social life?

Questionnaire for the Caregiving Family

You may also wish to gauge the emotional well-being of other family members. You can ask your family these questions.

1. Do they often feel neglected?
2. Are there frequent arguments in your home?
3. Do members of your family avoid coming home?
4. Are they moody and withdrawn?
5. Do they avoid inviting friends home?
6. Are they resorting to the use of drugs or alcohol?
7. Has your relationship become strained?
8. Do they refuse to accept the new, ill person as part of the family?

All responses for both the caregiver and caregiving family should be "no." If you or a member of your family answers "yes" to a few questions, call a family meeting to discuss these problems. Stating your problem and getting it into the open is the first step toward solving it. If you or a family member has answered with more than just a few "yes" responses, you will need the assistance of family counseling and perhaps will have to revise your living arrangements.

▶ PROMOTING INDEPENDENCE FOR YOUR PATIENT (AND YOURSELF)

Keeping your patient as independent as possible might not seem important at first, but the more independent your patient, the less dependence there will be upon you and your family. Promoting independence and self-care also improves self-esteem and self-worth. Your main goal is that your patient is as comfortable and independent as possible. The patient confined to a wheelchair, for instance, can still help with bathing. Also, the wheelchair can be rolled to the kitchen table, and the patient can pare and chop vegetables for the evening meal. He may even be able to push himself outside and up the sidewalk to visit a neighbor or watch a local team play baseball.

Willingness to remain independent differs with each patient. Some react to an illness by trying to be as independent as possible, while others want to become totally dependent upon their family. Encourage your patient to be as independent as physical and mental capacities allow.

Realize the patient may perform tasks slowly. For example, you can dust the living room tables in ten minutes, while your patient takes 30 minutes. Be patient while he performs this task, and praise his accomplishment. For the stroke victim with limited finger dexterity, it is very gratifying to finally be able to comb his hair without assistance. Encourage your patient to perform small tasks and some self-care.

Perhaps your patient would like to visit an old friend living in the same town. Drive the patient there, promising to return at a designated time. Other members of the family can also help promote independence. If a son, grandson, niece, or nephew offers to take your patient out, encourage this if health conditions permit.

A word of caution: Do not expect all family members to be eager to stay with or take out your patient for a few hours. Perhaps when you first mentioned to close relatives (excluding those of your immediate household) that Uncle Joe was coming to live with you, many offered their help. Now you find, however, that Cousin Jane is too busy with her own family, and your brother Tom finds one excuse after another not to lend a hand. Avoid being discouraged about this attitude or allowing it to break the bonds of friendship with these family members.

It is easy to see how some caregivers slip into the role of a martyr. Due to the circumstances of their patient's condition, they find themselves completely devoted to their patients. Although this complete devotion sounds admirable, these caregivers lose their own identity by not providing themselves with activities away from their patients. Ties with family and friends are severed due to this devotion, and the martyrs' world revolves only around their patients. Martyrs continually remind themselves that they are strong and can carry the burden alone.

This situation, however, becomes very sad for both patient and caregiver. Not only does the caregiver need a life of his/her own, but the patient will also benefit from having contact with other persons. It is possible that the martyr will become sick and no longer be able to care for the patient. Then the patient will have a long, difficult adjustment to new persons and surroundings. If the patient has to go to a nursing home or dies, the martyr caregiver finds him- or herself completely lost without friends, family, or social attachments. Stop and ask yourself if you are becoming a martyr.

Planning Time Away from Your Patient

You are not expected to, nor should you, spend 24 hours a day, seven days a week with your patient. Continue to participate in many of the activities outside the home you took part in before your patient came to live with you. Perhaps your patient is well enough to leave alone for a few hours while you attend your Wednesday bridge game or another regular activity. If not, perhaps a family member will stay with him during that time.

If neither of these alternatives is possible, consider hiring a companion for your patient. There is probably a responsible neighbor willing to do this, but you must also expect to pay this person a reasonable rate. A local employment agency or the Area Agency on Aging can be of assistance, but always insist on references, and do check references by telephone.

If your family spends the first two weeks of June at a summer cottage every year, plan to take your vacation as scheduled. After all, you still need a vacation. Consider hiring a companion for your patient for these two weeks, or investigate other alternatives. Boarding homes and nursing homes room patients on a weekly basis. A boarding home cares for patients who are fairly independent, while a nursing home cares for the more acutely ill. Boarding homes are usually less expensive.

Investigate these facilities in your neighborhood. Visit them first, and then have your patient visit if possible. Speak with other families whose loved ones reside there. Be certain to make all arrangements well in advance, and also be certain the temporary caregivers understand all areas of your patient's care, including diet, medications, and physical and mental limitations. Leave telephone numbers where you can be reached in case of an emergency, too.

Day care centers for the elderly can also be an alternative in planning a few hours away from your patient. Some nursing homes now provide such centers. This type of care is a spin-off of day care centers for infants and children. The patient is taken there at a specific time in the morning and stays a set number of hours. Lunch is provided, and many special activities are planned. Your patient will look forward to an outing at a day care center. Plan this as often as your budget allows, although the cost may be fairly expensive.

Other members of your immediate household should be instructed on proper care and should tend to your patient at times in the event that you become ill or have to leave the home for an extended time. They should be confident in all areas of care, such as preparing meals, giving a bath, toileting, and preparing and giving medications. Make special notes about diet; list telephone numbers of physician, pharmacy, and home medical supplier; write dates of upcoming doctor's and other appointments; and make sure family members know where to find this information.

Community Resources

Many communities have social centers for the elderly, and if your elderly patient's condition permits, he should visit this center. The main activity of the day usually takes place around the noon meal. It might be impossible to drive your patient to the community center daily, but attending once a week would do much to raise the patient's spirits and maintain communication with others of the same age. Van or bus service is provided in some areas.

Be sure not to overlook church and local organizations as resources. Everyone wants to feel needed and worthwhile. An elderly woman may become very involved with knitting lap robes for nursing home patients or making special favors for hospital patients. A man with a chronic illness may spend hours cutting wooden blocks or large wooden puzzles for the children in an orphanage.

The telephone book is a good source of information. Review the listings of human services provided in your area. Your county probably has a special program for the aging as well as a program for the younger, chronically ill person. In such programs they will evaluate your situation, and if needed, provide nurse's aides, homemakers, social workers, and chore workers either free of charge or for a minimal fee.

If your patient suffers with diabetes, cancer, or respiratory disease, look for the local chapters of these organizations and others in your phone book. (See also Appendix C.)

Depending upon your patient's condition, the physician may recommend that a home health nurse visit. Besides the nurse, some home health agencies also provide speech therapists, occupational therapists, home health aides, social workers, and physical therapists for in-home visits.

A skilled nurse will assess the patient's overall condition checking heart rate, blood pressure, lung function, and response to medications. Nursing skills also include wound and dressing care, drawing blood, injections, and health teaching. A physical therapist sets up an exercise program for your patient and assists with walking, and special equipment such as canes, and walkers. An occupational therapist assists with finer muscle activities such as eating and dressing.

Home health aides perform bathing and personal care. A social worker evaluates your home situation and makes referrals to other agencies as needed. These agencies include homemakers, the food stamp program, and transportation services. Other referrals may include family and marriage counseling, mental health counseling, and drug and alcohol programs. A social worker can also assist with financial information and referrals such as Medicare, Black Lung, Social Security, and Medical Assistance.

Hints for the Caregiver

Following is a list of hints to promote the emotional and physical well-being of the caregiver.

1. Take time for yourself daily.
2. Do not ignore your family and friends.
3. Pay attention to your own appearance.
4. Take one day at a time and one task at a time.
5. Care for your own physical and mental health.
6. Pace your activities.
7. Keep a happy attitude toward your patient, your family, and yourself.
8. Practice the same courtesy and politeness with your patient and family as you would with a guest in your home.
9. Use humor.
10. Be socially active.

11. Join support groups.
12. Invite friends to your home.
13. Encourage other members of your immediate family to help care for your patient.
14. Employ companions to care for your patient when needed.
15. Look to community organizations for further support and assistance.
16. Take pride in your accomplishments and do not become overwhelmed by disappointments.

▶ WHEN HOME CARE BECOMES IMPOSSIBLE

Sometimes it becomes impossible to care for your patient at home. Difficult problems could develop for you, your family, or your patient. Perhaps the patient's condition has deteriorated to such a degree that you can no longer give adequate care. On the other hand, your patient could be unhappy living in your home. Perhaps you are dissatisfied with your social life and feel too "tied down." Possibly your spouse or children feel neglected.

Now you will have to look into alternative means of care for your patient. A social worker can inform you about special care facilities in your area. Your alternatives will depend upon the patient's actual physical and mental condition. Boarding homes are available if your patient can perform some self-care. Domiciliary homes are available in some areas. These are foster homes in which surrogate families or caregivers take fairly independent individuals into their own homes to provide minimum assistance. However, if your patient's physical or mental condition is such that he is dependent upon others for care, a nursing home is your only alternative. Discuss these alternatives with your doctor.

If your patient does have to leave your home for whatever reason, do not consider this move a failure. If all involved tried their best to adapt to the living arrangements, there are no failures. Your love for each other has not changed and your patient knows you have tried. The agreement was for a specified trial period, and that period has ended.

CHAPTER 2

GETTING STARTED

▶ INFORMATION GATHERING

The question of what to do about an ill family member usually arises as a result of an accident or a rapid decline in that person's health. Your loved one is hospitalized at the present time, and you feel overwhelmed. There is so much to do in such a short time before bringing your patient home, and you do not know where to start.

First, you will have to know your patient's condition. Your patient could suffer from a wide range of illnesses, such as heart disease, stroke, or Alzheimer's disease. You need to know about any special diets, activity restrictions, and medications. No one is expecting you to suddenly become a medical expert. Relax. Take your time. Eventually you will gather all the information needed to give proper care. Besides, knowledge of the anatomy of the heart is not a requirement for giving good home health care to a heart patient.

Your best sources of information are the physician and nurses now caring for your patient. During visits to the hospital be observant of how others care for your family member, and do ask questions. No matter how trivial the question seems now, it may save both you and your patient much anguish and worry in the future. Make a list of the questions you want to ask your patient's doctor.

1. Is your patient allowed to walk up the stairs? (Your home is two stories, and the bathroom is upstairs.)
2. Will a hospital bed be needed? What about a wheelchair?
3. Is the physician assigning visiting nurses to come to your home after your patient is discharged from the hospital?
4. What about medications?
5. Will you need to prepare special meals for your patient?

The nurses at the hospital will review your patient's medications with you; the dietitian will give advice on special diets; the physical therapist will provide instructions on special exercises. Do not hesitate to question anyone at the hospital. They are professional persons who are concerned about your patient's welfare. They will answer all your questions, no matter how basic.

You will be absorbing a great deal of information from many sources, and soon you may find your mind is boggled with facts. Therefore, it will be helpful to take notes. Do not be ashamed to keep a written record of facts you want to remember, for this does not imply a lack of intelligence, but rather proves you care. All medical specialists, including physicians, nurses, and physical therapists, have an exasperating habit of using medical terms that are not familiar to the average person. You might think they speak in their medical terminology to keep you from understanding, but this is not true. The medical terms are so much a part of their lives that these specialists eventually assume everyone knows the jargon. Hopefully, you feel comfortable talking with your patient's physician. If your physician uses words you do not understand, stop him immediately and ask him to rephrase what he just said in terms you can understand. In a few months you will find yourself so familiar with medical terms that some of them become household words in your home.

Before your patient leaves the hospital, have a precise list of all medications (including doses and times to be taken), sample diet menus, and special exercises. You will feel much more confident about administering care if you have notes and written plans for reference after your patient comes home.

If climbing stairs is not allowed and you live in a two-story home, your first decision is which room to select for the sickroom. Access to a bathroom is an important consideration. If your patient is using a portable bedside commode (a chair frame with a toilet seat and a removable pail beneath) while in the hospital, you may decide to purchase one to use at home. The hospital bed your patient is now using is low to the floor, making it easier to get in and out of bed and also adjusting to many positions for comfort. You may need to obtain a hospital bed for home care.

Before your patient is discharged from the hospital, visit a local home medical supply company. You will be amazed at the items available for home care. The medical supply company staff can offer advice about equipment, handle the billing to insurance and Medicare, and deliver the items to your home.

Medicare pays as much as 80 percent of the cost of renting such equipment as a hospital bed, but not everyone who decides to use a hospital bed and who belongs to Medicare can rent one. Qualifications depend on your patient's medical problems and needs. Ask your physician about equipment you will need because a written physician's prescription is needed for items rented or purchased through Medicare. There is also a yearly deductible to be met.

If your patient cannot rent a bed from Medicare, yet you feel one is needed, check with local civic organizations who lend medical equipment. This equipment may be free, or perhaps the organization will ask for a small donation. Some health insurances help pay for home medical equipment. Veterans should inquire at the local Veterans Administration. The Easter Seal Society also rents equipment. Consider these and any other possible sources of help in obtaining equipment necessary for your patient's home care.

▶ FACTORS TO CONSIDER IN SELECTING A SICKROOM

Some changes to your home will be necessary, but these need not be drastic. You must first decide which room will be the most convenient for your patient's sickroom. There will be major changes if a spare bedroom is not available or if your patient has no access to that room. You may have to convert a den into your patient's room, but the rest of your home will require only minimal changes, such as the addition of ramps and safety railing.

The room used for your patient will depend on the physical layout of your home and on your patient's specific needs.

If you live in a typical, older two-story home, it is probably rather small. It has a living room, kitchen, and dining room on the first floor and three bedrooms and a bath upstairs. Your dining room is close to the kitchen, but the traffic pattern of the home diverts most visitors away from that area. For the time being, you decide your dining room is ideal for your patient's sickroom. When (and if) he is able to mount the stairs, your spare upstairs bedroom can be used.

If you live in a one-story home, selecting the room for your patient will not be too difficult. You can select a spare bedroom or a den. If your home has a finished recreation room in the basement with a bathroom nearby, this may be the ideal room for your patient. Remember, however, that most elderly persons have at least a touch of arthritis, and a damp basement may aggravate the condition.

Lighting

Sources of both artificial and natural lighting are a must. Your dining room used as a sickroom may contain one chandelier suspended over the table. An overhead ceiling light can be very tiresome and glaring to a person who has to spend a good deal of time in bed. If your chandelier does have a dimmer switch, it will be of some use, but you will need to install a table lamp next to the hospital bed. Night-lights will be needed in your patient's room. If he is able to use the bathroom, you will need one there, too. Use a night-light in any dark hallway your patient may have to walk through.

Electrical Supply

The greater number of electrical outlets that are available in the sickroom the better. If you select an electrical hospital bed because your patient can operate the controls and change the position of the bed himself, this requires a grounded outlet. Because of the potential fire hazard, refrain from using any extension cords, using grounded outlets instead. The table lamp also requires an outlet, and if you plan to have a television installed in the room, an outlet will be needed for that, too.

Depending on your patient's condition, even more electrical outlets may be needed. For example, a patient with a machine that produces oxygen (called an oxygen concentrator), will need an outlet for this special equipment. You may have to hire an electrician to install more electrical outlets or change the older outlets to three-pronged grounded outlets. (More about special equipment is discussed in Chapter 11.)

Privacy

Your patient may have been accustomed to living alone in a quiet home environment for years, and now he must adjust to living with your family. For this reason, every means of assuring some privacy must be used. If the dining room is used as a sickroom and is not equipped with a door, perhaps a folding wooden door can be installed. A curtain can give privacy, but this will not lessen noises from other rooms. Because your patient will also be using the bedside commode in this sickroom, a screen to enclose the commode for added privacy is desirable. Such a screen can be purchased, or perhaps a family member can build one. Suspending a rod from the ceiling and hanging a shower curtain also provides privacy and is less costly.

Select a room that is fairly quiet and away from the hustle and bustle of your family's routine if possible. To ensure even more privacy, blinds should be added to all windows. Also consider the view your patient will see since he may spend some time sitting by the window. A bird feeder placed outside the window can also give your patient many hours of enjoyment.

Water and Plumbing Supplies

If you use the dining room as the patient's room, the fact that it is located near the kitchen will not only be helpful with meals, it will also save many steps to the nearest sink for bathing and drinking water. The bedside commode, however, poses another problem. For cleanliness and the prevention of odors, the commode should be emptied after each use, so you will need to carry the pail beneath the commode to the bathroom each time it is to be emptied.

Another factor to consider is bathing. Until your patient's condition improves enough for him to walk up the stairs to a bathroom if necessary and to get in and out of a bathtub, sponge bathing will have to be done at the bedside.

Room Size

Your patient's sickroom should be fairly large, about 12 feet by 12 feet, and after excess furniture is removed, there should be plenty of room to place the bed where it can be used from either side. Placing one side of the bed against the wall makes it difficult to change linens and to assist your patient while he is lying in bed. You will also need a dresser or chest for your patient's personal items such as clothing, books, and so forth. A few photographs and other personal items from his former home will help to make the new room more homey. What a pleasant surprise it will be for your patient when he sees that his new room has a few reminders of the past. A prized piece of furniture such as a desk or small bookcase from his old home could be placed in the sickroom, but do avoid overcrowding this room with furniture.

Ventilation and Heating

Your patient may tend to become cold easily. The sickroom should be free of drafts, with windows that open to provide a breeze on suitable days. You will also want to air out the room periodically.

If the air in the sickroom is dry, a humidifier can be used. Conversely, if the air is humid, a dehumidifier may be needed.

Floor Covering

A nonslip linoleum is the best floor covering for a sickroom because it is easy to clean, and once your patient starts walking, a carpet will make walking more difficult. You may have spent hours waxing and buffing your floor, proud of the glossy finish, but an ill, weak person who must negotiate each step with caution will find that your waxed shine resembles an ice skating rink. For his safety, put beauty aside and strip all wax from the floor. Scatter rugs should also be removed because they are the culprit of many accidents of the ill.

Safety Devices

The patient who has difficulty walking will feel more confident with handrails along stairs and long halls. Those able to use the bathroom will need rails (grip bars) around the commode, bathtub, and shower. The patient prone to wandering about at night will need bed rails installed on the hospital bed. Bed rails (side rails) are useful for turning your patient in bed, too. Most patients are able to grasp the rail and help turn themselves onto their side.

If your patient is only able to walk a few feet or is confined to a wheelchair, install some ramps. Because most homes have a few steps from street level to the front porch, you will need a ramp here. Two sturdy planks will do. You can also edge the sides of the ramp with two-by-fours to make the ramp safer by eliminating the danger of the wheelchair slipping off the sides.

Also examine the areas your wheelchair patient will be negotiating inside the house. Measure the widths of doors and doorways to assure that a wheelchair will pass through them easily.

Furnishings

So far, your patient's room contains a hospital bed, chest, television, and table lamp. A table or bedside stand will be needed near the bed for easy access, preferably with some storage area. Your patient will be using a wheelchair when possible, but you should also plan to place a low, comfortable easy chair in the room.

If the ill person already had a favorite recliner, bring it to your home for his use. The physical therapist at the hospital can also assist you with selecting the proper chair. It should be sturdy and your patient should be able to get in and out of it without difficulty. Because a recliner is equipped with a footstool, it can be used to elevate your patient's legs. Swelling of the lower legs and feet is a problem for most elderly persons and also a problem for younger chronically ill persons if their circulation is poor. Elevating the feet and legs will help relieve this problem. A recliner also adjusts to several comfortable positions. Another chair should be installed near the recliner for visitors' use.

Your patient may require some special considerations in the choice of a chair. For the patient recovering from a fractured hip, a soft chair may not provide enough support, and it may be difficult to arise. Be sure to discuss the selection of chairs with your patient's physical therapist or physician.

Because clutter is the cause of many accidents, keep the sickroom as clutter free as possible. Too many sickrooms quickly become over-crowded with cardboard boxes of old books and hope chests full of family heirlooms. Soon there is nothing more than a narrow pathway. Pity the ill person who lives in a cluttered, crowded room. He is probably a little dizzy and unsteady when standing, has blurred vision and is perhaps learning to walk with a walker. If he must learn to negotiate through the maze in his room, is it any wonder this person might have an accident?

Use of a wheelchair also affects space in the patient's room. Turning a wheelchair around takes up a good deal of space, and this must be considered when arranging the furniture.

Your furniture need not be expensive. A card table will be fine to use in the room, and you will not have to worry about spills or marring the finish. Plastic, stackable storage boxes available at discount depart-ment stores can be used for a bedside stand and for storing bathing equipment and linens. Folding TV trays are also handy. They can be placed by your patient's recliner and can be folded to store out of the way when not needed.

Improvise with the pieces of furniture you now have. You will be pleased to see how easily your sickroom takes shape. (See Figure 1.)

▶ Personal Equipment

Unless your physician specifically orders some special equipment be-sides the basic hospital bed and other furniture you now have in your sickroom, do not worry about other items. You do not need every conceivable piece of equipment waiting for your patient's arrival. However, a banner that says "Welcome Home," or a vase of flowers can truly add a welcoming, personal touch.

Eventually you will gather the proper equipment needed for your patient, but trying to purchase a supply of items you think you might need will only lead to waste. Most of the personal items your patient now has in the hospital will suffice for the first few days at home.

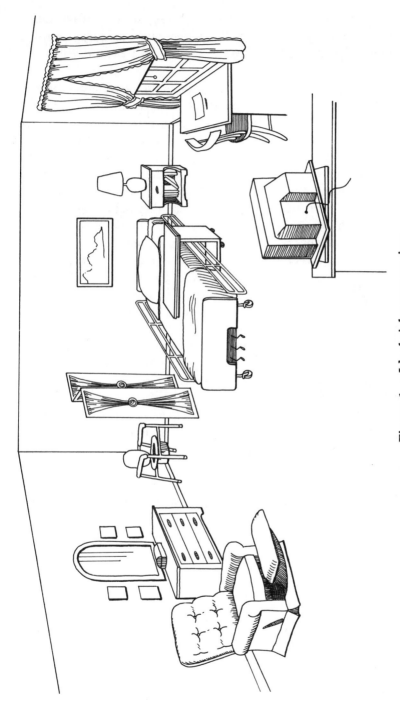

Figure 1. Ideal sickroom setting.

Just think of the everyday items you use, such as comb, brush, toothbrush, and mouthwash. If your patient wears dentures, he probably already has a supply of denture cream and a denture cup at the hospital.

Most hospitals now provide each patient with a variety of bathing and personal items that are disposable and used only for that patient. Consult the nurse. Usually you may take these items home. The washbasin, emesis basin (a small kidney-shaped basin useful to spit into while teeth brushing and rinsing the mouth), and bedpan are some of the items the hospital may allow the patient to take home when discharged. These items are plastic, yet durable, and in most hospitals the patient is charged for these disposable items. If you choose not to take these items home, they will be tossed into the garbage since the hospital cannot use them for another patient.

If your patient has been using a special pad on the hospital bed to help prevent bedsores, such as a sheepskin pad, an egg crate mattress pad, or heel protectors, ask about this, too. If your patient has been charged for these items, he is permitted to take them home. (These items are discussed in Chapter 4.)

If your patient has poor urine or bowel control, the hospital nurse has probably been using disposable plastic bed savers (also called incontinence pads or linen savers). Because most patients are charged for an entire package of these disposable pads, you may be permitted to take the remainder of an opened package home. Hospital policy will vary on these items, but do not hesitate to inquire in order to save some money.

Bathing, Washing, and Hair Care Needs

You will need some supplies for bathing and washing the patient. A few hair care supplies will also be necessary. Your list will include many of the following items:

1. Washbasin
2. Soap and soap dish (any good deodorant or moisturizing soap)
3. Washcloths, hand and bath towels
4. Denture cream, mouthwash, denture cup, and emesis basin

5. Deodorant and cosmetics (shaving supplies for males)
6. Face and body lotion, dusting powder, or cornstarch
7. Comb and brush
8. Shampoo (a dry shampoo used without water is handy)
9. Hair rollers for females
10. A hand mirror.

Clothing

Nightgowns. For female patients a nightgown should supply warmth yet be easy to slip into. If your patient (male or female) has to spend a good deal of time in bed, a gown that opens the entire length of the back will make using the bedpan and giving back care easier. These gowns are available at a hospital supply store, or you can easily open the back of any nightgown and apply a few ties for closures. Male patients will likely choose pajamas; however, for those who are not strictly confined to bed but have problems with buttons and zippers, soft, easy to wash jogging suits may be worn. Select robes that are warm and roomy.

Shoes and/or Slippers. Unless the physical therapist has recommended a specific type of shoe, such as a sturdy oxford in the case of a stroke patient, any patient would benefit from the use of an inexpensive pair of washable canvas jogging shoes with a nonskid sole. Shoes should always have low heels.

Stockings. The female should not wear garters because they restrict the circulation of blood in the legs. Ankle-high, knee-high, and thigh-high stockings are also too restrictive. Plain white cotton socks are best for both males and females.

Special elastic stockings may be ordered by the physician for the patient who has problems with blood clots (thrombophlebitis), and you should learn proper care and application of these stockings.

Underwear. The underwear worn by your patient depends on preference and need. Although it is not necessary that a female patient wear a bra, if she feels more comfortable with one, her wishes should be respected. Some women feel more comfortable in a woman's knitted undershirt. The patient with urinary or bowel problems will find that wearing panties or undershorts makes using the bedpan and bedside commode more difficult.

Other clothing. Bed jackets, sweaters, and shawls may be worn over nightgowns for added warmth. Some patients, especially women who wear nightgowns, find that knitted leg warmers are especially nice to keep the lower legs and arthritic knees warm. Specially made clothing, such as wrap-around dresses with Velcro® closures for females, and slacks and shirts with Velcro® closures for males are available at medical supply houses. A seamstress could adapt some of your patient's clothing to specific needs for ease of dressing and undressing. Choose clothing that is comfortable, washes easily, and requires no ironing.

Bed Linens

Mattress Covers. Easy-care mattress pads will be needed. Most hospital bed mattresses are equipped with a covering that is easily washed. Rubber mattress protectors, such as those used in baby's cribs, can be used also.

Fitted Sheets, Top Sheets, and Pillow Cases. Choose sheets and pillow cases in fabrics that are easy to care for and soft to the skin. Never starch sheets or pillow cases. Flannel sheets offer both warmth and softness.

Lift Sheets. Lift sheets or turning sheets are regular sheets folded and placed beneath the patient from mid-back to mid-thighs. These are helpful in turning the patient from side to side, and in the case of the patient who has poor urinary control, they sometimes save changing the entire bottom sheet.

Blankets. Any blanket that provides warmth will do, but NEVER USE AN ELECTRIC BLANKET on a senile patient or one who has poor control of urine or bowels. If your patient uses oxygen equipment, do not use a wool blanket because it could cause a spark.

Pillows. Several bed-size pillows will be needed, and at times a smaller pillow will be helpful with positioning your patient in bed or giving support to a limb. Waterproof pillow covers are also available.

▶ OTHER EQUIPMENT

Any other equipment will depend on your patient's situation and needs. For example, if your patient is able to use the bathroom, there is a variety of rails, safety equipment, and raised toilet seats available. Imagine how painful it must be for a patient who has just had hip surgery to lower himself to a standard commode. For these persons or ones suffering with severe arthritis of the knees and hips, a raised toilet seat is most helpful (see Figure 2).

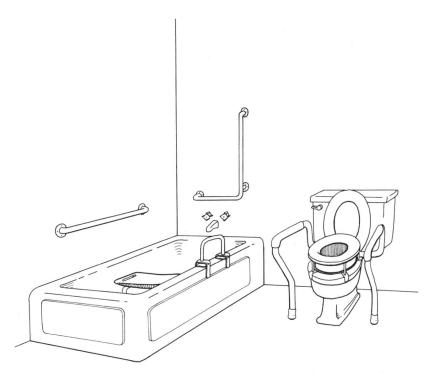

Figure 2.   Bathroom safety equipment including a raised
toilet seat.

If your patient is permitted to climb stairs, a sturdy handrail should be installed along one side of the stairs. Besides the local home medical supply house, mail-order companies can be helpful as a source for such equipment. (A list of mail-order catalogs is provided in Appendix B.)

Call Bells. A call bell is another necessary item for your patient's room as it is imperative that your patient have some sort of system for reaching you. This can be a simple cow bell (the type used at football games), a New Year's Eve-type noisemaker, or a sophisticated electronic system available at a local electronics shop. Whatever your system, test it to be certain it can be heard throughout your home. Nothing is more frightening to an ill person than awakening with pain in the middle of the night and not being able to call out for help.

Miscellaneous Equipment

In addition to personal equipment previously mentioned, a number of miscellaneous items can be invaluable to the caregiver. Following is a list of such items.

1. Thermometers may be oral or rectal. A rectal thermometer should be used for the patient who is mentally confused and could bite an oral thermometer. If your patient is using oxygen on a routine basis, you will also want to use a rectal thermometer because he tends to breathe through his mouth. The new digital, battery operated thermometers are easy to read with no fear of breakage.
2. Disposable hand wipes
3. Over-the-bed tray table
4. Water pitcher, glass, and straw
5. Bath scales
6. Calendar
7. Clock (a timer may be helpful for medicine schedules)
8. Night-light
9. Room deodorant spray
10. Disinfectant for cleaning bedside commode, bedpan, and general cleaning
11. Trash can with disposable liner

12. Heel protectors
13. Elbow protectors
14. Disposable rubber gloves
15. Adult disposable diapers
16. Disposable incontinence pads (bed savers, linen savers).

Emergency Equipment

The following emergency equipment should also be kept handy:

1. Flashlight
2. List of emergency telephone numbers posted at the telephone, including physician, ambulance, fire, police, home medical supply store, and poison control center
3. First aid booklet
4. Smoke alarms
5. Fire extinguishers.

Daily Diary

It will be very helpful if you keep a loose-leaf or spiral notebook of facts to remember about your patient. List pertinent information daily, such as medications, weight, and diet. You will then have a written record for reference as needed.

▶ ITEMS NOT TO USE

Heating Pads and Hot Water Bottles.   Heating pads and hot water bottles should be used on the elderly with extreme caution because their skin is less sensitive to heat and they could easily burn. If your patient insists upon using a heating pad, make certain the setting is on low and NEVER allow your patient to lie directly on top of it. Instead, lay the pad over the affected area.

For example, if your patient has back pain, turn him onto his side and position the pad over his back. Remove the pad at intervals and inspect the skin for any sign of burning or redness.

Razors. If your patient is taking a medication to thin the blood (blood thinners or anticoagulants), he is prone to bleeding easily and should be shaved with an electric shaver instead of a razor.

▶ PLANNING THE DAY

Your patient is home. His arrival has caused no problems because you had his room prepared and did some planning in advance. You have a copy of the hospital discharge summary, and the hospital nurse and/or physician reviewed each area carefully with you prior to discharge. The hospital discharge summary should list such information as diet, physical activities allowed or limited, medications, and other pertinent facts. (See Figure 3.)

The elderly feel more secure on a schedule. As the primary caregiver, you want everything to run smoothly for your patient, yourself, and your family. Therefore, you must plan a general time schedule of necessary tasks.

You know medications are to be given at scheduled times. Probably you have decided it would be convenient to prepare the patient's breakfast while you are preparing breakfast for the rest of the family. Plan to help bathe your patient after other family members have left for school and work each morning.

However, you may have to adapt your schedule to your patient's needs and wishes. The person who is accustomed to bathing before retiring each night may feel threatened if you try to change his routine. If bathing in the evening does not disrupt you or your family's schedule, be flexible and bathe your patient in the evening.

When planning your patient's morning routine, think about your own. As soon as you get out of bed in the morning, you use the toilet, wash your hands and face, and brush your teeth. Your patient's routine will undoubtedly be similar. Therefore, before starting breakfast in the morning, check on your patient. Ask if he slept well, if he is comfortable, or if he is having any pain. If any medications are to be given before breakfast, they may be given at this time. Then you can assist your patient with using the toilet. Depending upon his condition, this will either be done at the bed, using the bedside commode, or in the bathroom (see Chapter 3).

After toileting, your patient can then wash his hands and face and brush his teeth. If he is confined to bed, adjust the bed to a sitting

Sunny Place Hospital
Sunny Lane
Philipsburg, Pa.

DISCHARGE SUMMARV

Ryan, Catherine
100100 T. Harvey
89764564 092486

Activities:

No climbing stairs
Rest frequently with feet elevated

Diet:

No added salt

Medications:

Digoxin 0.125 mg one tab. twice a day
Hydrochlorothiazide 50 mg one tab daily
Nitroglycerin 10 cm skin disk one to skin daily
Nitroglycerin tab. gr ½oo under tongue every 5
*   minutes as needed for chest pain X 3*
Multivitamin one tab. daily
Docusate Sodium cap. 2 at hour of sleep
Milk of Magnesia 3 Tbsp. hour of sleep
*   as needed*

Special Instructions:

See physician at medical center in 2 weeks
Call for appointment
Weigh every AM and report 3 lb. weight gain

Signature of nurse

Signature of physician

C. Pearce RN

J. Harvey MD

Figure 3.   A hospital discharge summary.

position and place the equipment on the over-the-bed table. If your patient is able to get out of bed, he then may sit at the table in his room while you prepare and eat breakfast with your family.

After breakfast, you can assist your patient with bathing and personal care. When that is completed, you and your patient can have a mid-morning coffee or juice break together. Plan also to have lunch and dinner at a set time.

Schedule a quiet time each afternoon when the patient can rest, and give yourself some time to relax and rest, too. A nap is unnecessary; in fact, napping too long in the afternoon sometimes ruins a good night's sleep. However, do have your patient rest for at least an hour each afternoon, either in bed or in the recliner.

It is unnecessary for everyone in your home to go to bed at the same time, but designate a time each evening when all televisions, radios, and so forth are turned to a low volume. Before going to bed each evening, you and your patient can follow the same routine of toileting, hand washing, and teeth brushing as in the morning.

Set aside some time each day to be alone with your family, and also enable your patient to have some daily privacy. Although you want your loved one to feel wanted as a part of your family, your patient should respect you and your family's wish to have time alone together. In return, you should respect your patient's privacy by providing times when he is undisturbed. The patient should feel free to invite guests to his room and speak with them privately, and thus you should be free to have your own guests visit without interruption from your patient. Ground rules on respecting privacy should be agreed upon as soon as possible when your patient comes to live with you.

Example of a Daily Schedule

Following is a sample daily schedule that can guide you in making one to use with your patient.

7:30 A.M.	Awaken your patient. Assist with toileting, hand washing, and teeth brushing. Give any before breakfast medicine, if ordered.
7:40	Prepare breakfast.
8:00	Serve your patient breakfast in his room. (Have breakfast with your family.)

9:00	Bathe your patient. Change linens and care for room as needed. Give medications.
10:00	Have juice or coffee break with your patient.
12:00	Serve patient's lunch.
1:00 P.M.	Give medications, if ordered.
2:00	Rest for one hour (a quiet time with noise kept at a minimum).
5:00	Give medications, if ordered.
6:00	Serve dinner (your patient eats with you and your family if possible).
9:00	Have a quiet time (all TVs, radios, and so forth turned to low volume). Assist your patient with toileting, hand washing, and teeth brushing. Prepare patient for bed as needed. Give nighttime medications, if ordered.

Your schedule will be flexible, and of course, you will offer toileting, give juices and fluids, snacks, and medications as needed. This schedule is not as hectic as it seems; furthermore, you should designate other family members to help when possible. Go over your schedule with your patient and your family and make additional copies if needed.

Family Meetings

To help everyone adjust to your family's new living arrangements and to promote harmony, include family meetings as part of your new routine. Call family meetings as necessary, but avoid holding them at mealtime. At first, you, your patient, and your family may have to meet daily to solve any problems that develop. Announce your meetings and refer to them as "family meetings," so everyone in the household is aware that this is a special time to discuss problems in a calm and orderly manner.

Problems for discussion at these meetings may be simple or complex. Perhaps your teenager dislikes turning down the volume of the stereo at 9 P.M., or your patient is unhappy with his meals. Whatever the problem, it is best to face it and discuss it calmly before the problem becomes a trouble spot that causes anger and resentment. After a time, you will probably only call weekly or monthly family meetings as everyone adjusts to this new living situation.

CHAPTER 3

PROVIDING
PERSONAL CARE

▶ BATHING PROCEDURES

Now that your family has left for work and school, you are completely alone with your patient, and you feel a little timid. This is the time of the morning scheduled for your patient's bath, but even though you bathed your children when they were babies, you have never given a bath to an adult.

The skin is the largest organ of the body, and during the bath is the ideal time to observe your patient for any signs of skin problems. Most elderly persons tend to have dry skin, and contrary to beliefs that a daily bath is essential for cleanliness, it is unnecessary to give a complete bath every day. The legs and arms of the elderly are prone to dryness and scaling; therefore, an application of skin lotion or baby oil would be of more benefit than a daily scrubbing with soap and water.

Areas that do tend to perspire, such as the underarms, under the breast in heavier built females, and the genital and rectal area should be washed at least daily and more often if necessary. Some heavy females also have what is called an abdominal apron, a sagging of the abdomen over the groin area, and this should be cleansed daily because chaffing is common.

A guideline to follow is: Anywhere two skin surfaces touch, be especially cautious. One skin surface may irritate the other, and such an area is usually warm and moist, providing a good place for bacteria to grow. While bathing an obese patient, all skin folds (creases) should be inspected and cleansed daily.

Perhaps you have assumed that the only reason you are bathing your patient is to cleanse the body. However, the bath also stimulates the blood circulation, provides mild exercise, and promotes comfort.

To begin the bathing procedure, prepare your patient and the room for bathing. Adjust room temperature if necessary. Most older patients seem to notice the slightest drop in room temperature and will feel chilled, so you will probably want to turn up the thermostat a few degrees.

Of course, you will close all doors and blinds to assure privacy. This is also a convenient time to offer your patient the use of the toilet or bedside commode. Wash your hands before you start bathing your patient.

Assemble equipment and then recheck to make certain all items you need are included, thus avoiding wasted steps for a forgotten item. You will need a basin, soap, soap dish, towels, washcloth, skin lotion, deodorant, powder, a clean change of clothing, and a flannel blanket for warmth. Other items you may need, such as incontinence pads and adult disposable diapers, will depend on your patient's condition.

The bath water should range from 100° to 110° Fahrenheit. Check the temperature by holding your inner wrist or elbow in the water for a few seconds. If the water feels too hot for your skin, it is much too hot for the patient's delicate skin. Bath thermometers are also available for this purpose.

The type of bath you give will vary, depending on your patient's condition. All patients should be encouraged to assist with their own bathing as much as possible. Allowing your patient to bathe as much of his body as he is capable of increases confidence and self-esteem, besides proving mild exercise and stimulating the circulation.

Some embarrassment on your part will only be natural, and your patient will feel just as embarrassed, if not more so. To help you both feel more at ease, turn on the television or radio to add a little distraction. Talk with your patient while you work. The weather or the news you heard on the morning broadcast makes suitable discussion. This does not mean that you have to keep up a lively conversation while giving a bath, but talking will help you both relax.

The Partial Assist Bathing Procedure

Condition permitting, your patient can sit on the edge of the bed to wash his upper body. Place an incontinence pad under the buttocks to prevent bed and linens from becoming wet. Cover your patient's lower body with a flannel blanket to prevent chilling. If able, your patient can undress himself; if not, you will need to do this.

Undress your patient without undue bodily exposure by covering the lower body while removing the nightgown or pajama top. Never expose more of the body than necessary. A female can hold the flannel blanket lightly over her breasts while you remove first one arm from the sleeve of her nightgown, then the other arm, and finally her entire nightgown.

Your patient is ready to start bathing, and you can leave the room, condition permitting, while he washes and dries his face, neck, arms, hands, chest, and abdomen. If the patient is unable to bathe the rest of his body, you will help. When you return, ask him to lie on the bed so you can assist.

Covering your patient once more with the flannel blanket to prevent chilling, slip off the pajama bottoms or underwear by reaching beneath the blanket and asking him to lift his hips. You have removed the lower clothing without exposing the patient.

Now you are ready to bathe the legs. Uncover only one leg at a time. Spread the bath towel lengthwise, underneath the leg to protect the bed. To wash the back of the leg, gently bend the knee by placing your hand beneath the knee and applying gentle, upward pressure. Bathe and dry the leg using long, smooth strokes moving from ankle to hip. If uncertain whether you are being too gentle or using too much pressure, ask your patient, "Am I being too rough?" or "Would you like me to apply more pressure?" or "Is this comfortable for you?"

Lotion can then be applied, but do not massage the leg. This is especially important if your patient is prone to blood clots as rubbing the leg could dislodge a blood clot if one is present. After finishing with the first leg, cover it, proceeding with the other leg in the same manner.

When both legs are washed, dried, and lotioned, have your patient turn on his side while you wash his back and buttocks. Place the towel lengthwise over the bed along the back and buttocks, and tuck the edge beneath the back and buttocks. To prevent exposing and chilling your patient, cover the chest and legs with a flannel blanket while you bathe, rinse, and dry the back area. You are now ready to give a back massage.

The Back Massage. The back massage is soothing to your patient and allows you to give a little special attention. It also provides mild stimulation to the skin and helps circulation.

Any good hand or body lotion will be fine for your patient's back rub. However, the skin lotion is cold; to warm it, spread the lotion over your own hands and then rub them together before applying. The strength you exert while massaging the back will depend on your patient. Apply gentle pressure for the frail and thin female, but the muscular male patient will desire stronger pressure. Ask if the amount of pressure is comfortable.

Place your lotioned palms at the base of the spine (on either side of the spine but not directly over it) and massage upward, moving across the shoulders and returning with either palm at the sides of the back. Then using the balls of your fingers, massage the back and base of the spine with smooth, circular motions. The base of the spine (sacrum) is especially prone to bedsores. Apply more lotion as needed to allow your hands to glide easily. Massage the neck and shoulders, too. Use the towel to blot the excess lotion from your patient's back when the massage is completed. Now you are ready to continue with the bath.

The rectal area is washed next. You may wish to wear disposable gloves, especially if your patient has poor bowel or urinary control. Wash from the front to the back, so you do not introduce any bacteria from the rectal area into the urinary opening. Rinse and dry well.

Using clean water, your patient can wash the genital area. Condition permitting, you can leave the room at this time. Simply say, "I'll leave the room while you finish your bath," or "I'll wait outside until you wash between your legs."

When you return, you can help apply deodorant and dusting powder. Dusting powder or cornstarch is especially important where there are skin folds (creases) and two areas of skin touch, such as under the breast, abdominal aprons, and at the junction of the thighs and groin. A light dusting is all that is necessary. Too much powder will cause caking and lead to irritation.

Your patient can now be dressed before washing the feet. Use the same technique of covering him with the flannel blanket, so you do not expose him unnecessarily. Clean water will be needed for the rest of the bath, and the patient can sit on the side of the bed to soak his feet in the basin placed on the floor. On the other hand, you may move the patient to a chair, and place the basin on a footstool, so it is at a comfortable height.

Although it is good to soak the feet, they need not be soaked for a prolonged time. A few minutes is sufficient. Spread the toes, clean and inspect the areas between the toes, and dry well. Lotion may be applied to the feet, but dusting powder should be used between the toes to absorb moisture. Do not apply both lotion and dusting powder to the same area; this will cause caking.

Other Bathing Tips. The following suggestions will also be helpful to the caregiver.

1. The hands should be soaked in a basin of water at least weekly. This is a good time to observe the nails and give nail care if necessary.
2. Cornstarch works just as well as dusting powder, and it is less costly. Apply it with a powder puff, or put it in a shaker container, such as a large pepper shaker. (You may have to enlarge the holes of the container slightly.)
3. Change the bath water as needed if it becomes dirty or cool.
4. If water is spilled on the floor, wipe it up immediately to prevent falls.
5. Keep all radios and other electrical equipment away from the bathing area.
6. A good rule to follow is to bathe the area near you first and work to the other side. That is, bathe the arm near you and then the arm on the other side. Working in this manner will prevent jumping from one side of the body to the other, and your work will be more orderly.
7. When bathing the arms or legs, support them by placing your hand beneath the joint. Support the arm beneath the elbow and the leg beneath the knee. Support the foot by grasping the heel and ankle area.

Tips for the Caregiver. The comfort and protection of the caregiver should also be considered during the bathing procedure.

1. Cover any open cuts or wounds with a plastic adhesive strip and wear gloves to protect a cut on the hand.

2. Wear loose, comfortable clothing while bathing your patient; the temperature of the room will feel warm to you.

3. Wear comfortable, flat-heeled shoes.

4. To protect your own clothing, wear an apron.

5. If you feel more comfortable wearing disposable gloves during the entire bath, then by all means do so.

6. Wear disposable gloves if your patient has any skin rash or open, draining sores.

7. You may dry your own hands with the patient's towel during the bath, but when finished with the bath, wash your hands. Lather them well, rinse them under running water, and dry them on a clean towel or a paper towel.

8. Clean your nails frequently. It is best to keep them cut short.

The Complete Bed Bath Procedure

If your patient is unable to give any assistance with the bath, you will bathe him completely. The same principles apply as for the partial bath. Only expose the area to be bathed, and drape the towel to protect the bed as you work.

Before getting started, raise or lower the height of the bed to a comfortable working position for you. You want to bathe your patient without bending over and putting a strain on your back. Practice good posture by keeping your back straight and your body erect while you work. You are bound to suffer from backaches if you bend over the patient's bed constantly. Starting now, remind yourself to practice good posture and be kind to your own body as well as your patient's.

A complete bed bath really is not difficult. Actually, you do it all the time when you bathe yourself. True, you do not bathe yourself in bed using a basin of water, but the same techniques apply.

Elevate the head of the bed to a comfortable position for your patient. Assemble the same equipment as for the partial bed bath. An over-the-bed table is handy for this equipment. If you do not have an over-the-bed table, you can improvise by using a metal kitchen utility cart or an old stand. If you are afraid of damaging the table, protect the finish with a plastic cover.

Cover your patient with the flannel blanket and remove the night-gown or pajama top with the blanket in place as instructed for a partial bath. Drape a towel over your patient's chest and tuck it under the chin. Wash the face first. Using only plain water and NO soap on your washcloth, gently cleanse the eye area, working from the nose side outward. You may then use soap to gently wash the rest of the face. (Some women never use soap on their face, so ask first.)

Wring your washcloth well to gently wash the ears. Rinse and dry them well so no water or soap is left in the ear canal. Cotton-tipped applicators are not recommended for cleaning the ears.

Now move down to the neck area. Wash the front and sides of the neck now. Later, when your patient turns onto his side for you to wash his back, you can wash the back of the neck.

Next wash your patient's arms. Exposing the arm near you, drape the towel lengthwise beneath the arm and wash from the wrist to the shoulders, using long, smooth strokes. Wash the hand at this time. Simply bathe it with the washcloth, or place the basin on the bed and soak the hand for a short time. If you soak your patient's hand, be certain your basin is only about half full of water, and protect the bed with an incontinence pad. After you have washed, rinsed, and dried your patient's arm and hand well, apply lotion. When you have finished with that arm, cover it and bathe the other arm in the same way.

The chest or breast area is next. Wash the underarm area at this time and apply deodorant. Most women also like a light dusting of powder under their breasts.

Drape the towel over the chest while you wash, rinse, and dry the abdominal area. When finished, cover the chest and abdomen with the flannel blanket and bathe the legs. Proceed just as you did with the arms, working with the near one first.

If your patient is unable to sit at the side of the bed to soak his feet, place the basin on the bed (see Figure 1). Use a disposable bed protector under the basin to catch any splashing water, and be sure the basin does not contain so much water that it overflows when your patient's foot is inserted. Bend your patient's leg at the knee and place his foot in the basin. Be careful not to stretch or force the foot or leg, and only attempt to soak one foot at a time.

It seems like a bother to soak the feet in a basin on the bed, but to the bed patient, this is very comforting and relaxing. If your patient is uncooperative or has difficulty positioning his leg with his foot in the basin, simply bathe the foot area with a washcloth.

Next have your patient turn onto his side, and using clean water, proceed to wash the back, shoulders, back of the neck, and buttocks. Be certain your patient is comfortable in the side position, and place a

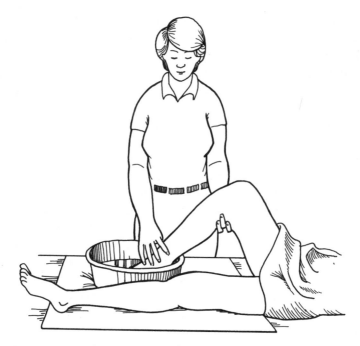

Figure 1.   Soaking the foot by placing a basin on the bed.

pillow under his head. Massage his back, buttocks, and hips with lotion.

If you prefer, wear disposable gloves to cleanse the rectal area. Always wash from the front toward the rectal area.

If your patient is severely ill or weak, which is probable since he is unable to bathe himself, you can change the bottom bed sheets at this time. This is only necessary if your patient cannot get out of bed to have it made. (The procedure for making an occupied bed is described later in this chapter.)

The entire back area has now been bathed, and the bottom bed sheets have been changed if necessary. Now help your patient turn over onto his back once more, and cleanse the genital area. Get clean water for this.

An uncircumcised male will need to have the foreskin of his penis gently pulled back for proper cleansing. After cleansing the tip of the penis, return the foreskin to its original position. The scrotum area should be cleansed gently and dried well. If you are a female, perhaps a male family member would be willing to bathe the genital area for you.

Bathe the female genital area by working from the front to back (rectal area), and use a clean section of the washcloth for each stroke. Pat dry. A light dusting of powder is fine, but use it sparingly. It is thought the powders applied to this area sometimes enter the urinary opening or vaginal area and cause infections. If you are a male, perhaps a female family member would bathe the genital area for you.

The proper sequence for the complete bed bath has just been described. Start with the eyes, face, neck, and ears. Next, wash the arms, hands, chest, and abdominal area. Then clean the legs, feet, back, buttocks, and rectal area. The genital area is last.

You have now given a complete bed bath and it probably was not as difficult as you imagined. The first time you bathed your new baby, you were anxious. With a little practice, however, it became part of your daily routine. The same is true with bathing an adult. After some practice you will be able to give a complete bed bath as well as any nurse. In fact, your bath will be better because your relationship with your patient is of a much more personal and loving nature.

Depending on whether you bathe your patient completely or just apply lotion to the dry skin areas such as arms and legs, some days it will take longer than others to bathe your patient. Do not be concerned if your first few bed baths are somewhat unorganized. After a few attempts you will become organized, learn exactly what equipment you need, and adapt the procedure to your specific patient.

The Tub Bath

Your patient may be physically able to take a tub bath. Many safety devices are available for patients who can get in and out of the tub. A sturdy bar may be installed along the wall of the tub for your patient to grip while getting in and out of the bath. This type of bar may be purchased at a local medical supply company, or you can make one from sections of cast-iron water pipe and elbows. Whether you make or purchase this equipment, it is important that the ends of the bar are fastened securely to a wall joist to assure adequate support. Bath seats, which extend across the width of the tub, are also helpful if your patient is not agile enough to be lowered completely into the tub.

A plain, straight-backed chair, such as a kitchen chair, should also be placed alongside the tub for your patient to sit on before entering the tub and after getting out. Place a flannel sheet over the chair for warmth.

Use a rubber bath mat inside the tub to prevent slipping, and place a heavy towel or mat on the floor outside the tub. DO NOT USE BATH OIL in the water because this makes the tub slick and increases the risk of falling.

Once you have assisted your patient into the tub, proceed with his bath, starting with the face and ending with the genital and rectal region. For easier access to the rectal region, it is better to wait until the finish of the bath when your patient is standing outside the tub. You may shampoo your patient's hair in the tub, but always provide a washcloth for him to place over his eyes during shampooing and rinsing.

When washing is completed, drain the water from the tub and begin to dry your patient while he is still sitting in the tub. Dry his hands especially well, so he can get a firm grip on the railing to assist with getting out of the tub. Help your patient out of the tub to the chair provided, and then wrap him with the bath sheet. Finish drying his body well, and apply powder and lotion as desired.

A tub bath can be very frightening to an ill person. If he is weak or extremely fearful, he may faint. In such cases it would be best to give a complete bed bath instead. If you do decide your patient's condition is strong enough to endure a tub bath, both you and he may feel more comfortable having a second person assist with getting him in and out of the tub. NEVER leave your patient alone while he is in the tub. Keep electrical equipment such as hair dryers away from the tub. Check the water temperature with your elbow or inner arm. Water that is too hot will naturally cause burning. Water that is bearable, yet just a little too hot, can also cause fainting.

The Shower Bath

Your patient may be able to take a shower bath. A special nonskid chair is available for the patient to sit on during the shower. Test this chair yourself before placing your patient on it. Also adjust the shower head. The spray of water should not hit directly on your patient's face or chest; it is better to direct the spray to the thigh or leg area. A shower head that swivels into different positions or a hand-held shower works well. Be sure to adjust the water temperature and check it constantly during the shower to protect your patient from scalding or chilling.

A kitchen chair can be placed outside the shower for your patient to sit on before and directly following the shower. Wrap the patient in the flannel sheet immediately following the shower to prevent chilling. Then apply lotion or powder as desired.

For your patient's safety, avoid using bath oil or baby oil because this could cause a slip or fall. Wipe up all water splashes around the shower stall before attempting to walk your patient from the area.

While assisting with a shower bath, you will not be able to close the shower curtain because you have to keep a constant surveillance on your patient and the water temperature. You will probably want to wear old clothing or a waterproof apron.

It is possible to give a shower to a patient confined to a wheelchair. If your shower is wide and the stall has a low rail along the floor, you can probably roll the wheelchair directly into the shower and let your patient shower sitting in the wheelchair. If this is not possible, set the wheelchair as close to the shower stall as possible and then help transfer your patient to the shower chair. Your patient will have to be able to bear some weight on his legs to move from wheelchair to shower chair. Have another person help with this, at least the first few times, until you are certain you can transfer your patient from wheelchair to shower chair and back to the wheelchair without assistance.

▶ Mouth care

Mouth care should be performed at least twice a day, morning and night, and more often if necessary. For example, some patients tend to hold food in their mouth for long periods of time, and they will need more frequent mouth care.

Teeth Brushing

If your patient wears dentures, brush or soak them as preferred using the emesis basin, denture cup, and water, and rinse well after soaking. Always encourage your patient to do as much personal care as possible. However, if he cannot clean his own dentures, you can take them to the sink to brush and rinse as necessary. The emesis basin is convenient for carrying them to the sink.

The patient with natural teeth can brush them at the sink or at the bedside. If you must brush your patient's teeth, brush gently taking care not to injure the gums. Disposable toothbrushes made of soft squares of spongy material attached to a stick are available to use once and throw away.

While assisting with teeth brushing, inspect your patient's mouth for sores. Check the gum line for signs of oozing pus, such as would be present with an abscessed tooth, and inspect the denture area for signs of irritation from ill-fitting dentures.

This is also the time to examine your patient's tongue. A thickly coated white or brown tongue usually means the patient is not drinking enough fluids. Clean this material from your patient's tongue by gently stroking with a piece of gauze dipped in a mixture of half water and half hydrogen peroxide. Wear disposable gloves to protect your hands from mouth secretions. It may take several applications to remove this coating. Encouraging more fluids and frequent mouth rinsing will help this condition.

CAUTION: If your patient is confused or combative, do not attempt to place your fingers in his mouth. Cotton-tipped applicators may also be used for mouth care, but if your patient is uncooperative, it is best to try again at another time.

Mouthwashes

Any good commercial mouthwash is suitable, but you can also use a solution of half water and half peroxide. Just be certain your patient does not swallow this solution. Salt water is also a soothing mouthwash and can be made by mixing one teaspoon of table salt to one quart of water. However, if your patient is on a low salt or salt free diet, do not use salt water.

▶ HAIR CARE

If your patient is able, encourage him to comb or brush his own hair. If you must comb your patient's hair, place him in a sitting position and drape a towel over his shoulders and pillow. Inspect the scalp for signs of sores, dandruff, or crusting. For the female patient with long hair, a spray detangler will be helpful. If her hair is tangled, work with a small section at a time, starting at the ends of the hair and gradually working toward the scalp. Style the hair as your patient desires.

Shampooing the Hair

For the very ill or weak patient it may be best to delay shampooing the hair until his condition is improved. A dry shampoo can be used for the very ill. Most elderly persons tend to have dry hair, and you need not concern yourself if you delay shampooing for a week or even two.

The patient who is able to stand can shampoo at the sink. If your patient cannot stand, he may sit on the edge of the bed and bend his head over a washbasin placed on the bedside stand or table. Proceed with caution, however, since this head-bent position may cause dizziness. You will need additional containers of water for this procedure. You may want the assistance of a family member.

Drape a towel over your patient's shoulders and allow him to place a washcloth over the eyes. You may also place cotton in the ear canals to prevent water from collecting in the ears.

If you have noticed crusting of the scalp (resembling cradle cap in babies), apply baby oil prior to the shampoo to loosen these crusts. Shampoo the hair as you would your own: wet the hair, apply shampoo, massage gently using your fingertips (not nails), and then rinse. Repeat the procedure with clean, warm water, and empty the basin as needed. Cream rinse may be used. Dry your patient's hair well or use a blow dryer after removing all water and wiping up all spills. Comb and style the hair as desired.

Most persons, especially females, are very particular about their hair. Not only does shampooing and styling provide comfort, but it also enhances your patient's self-esteem. Also consult beauticians in the area. Many are willing to tend to the shut-in patient; but of course, their fee will be a little higher for this service. Barbers are also willing to make home calls.

Shampooing the Bed Patient

Shampooing the patient strictly confined to bed is difficult. You will need assistance from other family members or perhaps from a beautician. An inflatable plastic shampoo basin is available for this purpose. The basin is positioned under the head, and the water is drained into a pail placed on the floor below the bed. During shampooing make sure your patient is comfortable, and pad and protect his neck from strain. An incontinence pad wrapped over a large bath towel can be used for this padding. Also protect the bed with incontinence pads.

▶ SHAVING PROCEDURES

The Male Shave

A facial shave promotes a man's comfort and enhances his appearance. For the patient who is able to shave himself, you need only assemble the equipment on the bedside table. This includes a basin of warm water, towel, mirror, safety razor, shaving cream, and after-shave.

However, if your patient is taking anticoagulants for a clotting problem, he is prone to bleeding, so an electric razor should be used. DO NOT use an electric razor, however, if your patient is using oxygen equipment.

If your patient is unable to shave himself, it is quite an easy procedure for you to shave his face with an electric razor. Be sure you have a good light and place your patient in a sitting position with the bed adjusted to a comfortable working height for you. Then drape a towel over his upper chest and shoulder area. An application of preshave will help remove oils from his skin. Using a circular motion with the razor, shave each area of the face and neck until it feels smooth to the touch. Then apply after-shave. Clean the razor head when finished.

Shaving with a safety razor is more difficult and requires some cooperation. Sudden movement may cause nicks, so your patient needs to hold his head still. Your patient can also help by puffing his cheeks and turning his head as needed. If you are a female caregiver, first ask a male family member to shave the patient while you observe. Then have him watch you shave your patient until you feel confident. If your patient is mentally confused or uncooperative, however, do not attempt at all to use a safety razor.

The Female Patient

Occasionally a female may have a few chin hairs or hair on her upper lip. This seems to develop with the aging process. Shave these areas with an electric razor as needed. She will appreciate your effort to keep her as attractive as possible. If you notice any coarse hairs growing from moles, do not shave this area. Instead, using small scissors, carefully clip the hair as close to the mole as possible. Never pluck hairs from moles.

▶ TOILETING ASSISTANCE

Helping your patient with toileting is not a difficult task. Your main concerns should be that the patient is comfortable, not unnecessarily exposed or embarrassed, and that privacy is respected as much as capabilities allow.

Always treat your patient with respect, and by the same token, always treat your patient's body with respect. Practice the art of empathy, putting yourself in your patient's place and being sensitive to his feelings and thoughts.

Wash your hands and have your patient do the same before toileting. If at all possible, your patient should be gotten out of bed to use the bedside commode or bathroom, instead of being placed on a bedpan or given a urinal. Your patient will assume a natural position for urinating or having a bowel movement while using the commode. On the other hand, using a bedpan or urinal in bed may cause difficulty with urinating or having a bowel movement due to the unnatural position. If you have ever had to use a bedpan, you know the unnatural feeling of having to sit or lie in bed to perform these functions.

Using the Bedside Commode and Toilet

Hopefully your patient will be physically able to use a bathroom toilet or a bedside commode. If your patient must use a bedside commode and you have not yet obtained one, make a substitute commode chair by placing the bedpan on a chair near the bedside. The chair should have sturdy arms and be protected from soiling.

The very weak or ill patient will need supervision even while using the bedside commode or bathroom toilet. If you are in doubt about his condition, for example, if he is dizzy, mentally confused, or experiencing pain or shortness of breath, then by all means stay with him. You may feel embarrassed about this at first, and so will your patient, but safety is your priority. You can say, "I'm your nurse now, and I'll stay with you just like the nurses did at the hospital," or "You're very weak. I'll stay with you so you don't fall." In a short time you will find that the embarrassment fades. After all, you are both adults, and the elimination of waste is a normal bodily function.

If your patient can be left alone while using the bedside commode or bathroom toilet, place a call bell within reach. You can purchase an extra call bell to keep in the bathroom or at the bedside commode.

Using a Bedpan or Urinal

If your patient is very ill or not able to get out of bed to use the bedside commode or bathroom, the urinal or bedpan can be used in bed with your assistance. Before placing a bedpan or urinal, close all doors to ensure privacy. The metal bedpan is usually cold, but it can be warmed by running hot water over it. Make certain the bedpan is not too hot to touch (metal does conduct heat), and dry it before placing it under your patient. Plastic bedpans which are not as cold, are more commonly used now.

Applying a light sprinkling of powder over the seat portion of the pan helps it slide under your patient's buttocks more easily. If your patient is very frail and thin, pad the seat portion of the pan with several folds of cloth or a piece of foam. A linen saver placed beneath the pan will catch any spills.

Besides the regular sized bedpan, a fracture bedpan is available (see Figure 2). It is smaller in size, and most persons find it easier to use. A very large individual may feel insecure using the fracture bedpan and fear that he will "overflow" the pan, although this rarely happens.

If your patient must remain in bed, elevate the head of the bed slightly before placing the pan. Then fold back the sheets and adjust the gown as necessary. Ask your patient to raise his hips. He will need to place his feet firmly on the bed and flex his knees in order to do this.

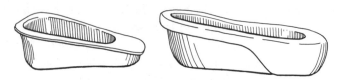

Figure 2.   A fracture pan and a regular bedpan. The smaller end of the fracture pan is placed beneath the patient's buttocks.

Slide the pan underneath the buttocks, making sure it is positioned correctly. Adjust the head of the bed to a higher sitting position, and be certain that your patient is comfortable. Elevate the side rails so your patient will feel more secure and will be able to adjust his position if necessary by grasping the rails. Provide toilet tissue and have the call bell within easy reach. Leave the room to give privacy if possible.

When your patient is finished with the bedpan, lower the head of the bed slightly. Ask him to once again raise his hips while you hold the pan securely. Slide the bedpan from under the buttocks, being careful not to drag it across the skin which could cause injury.

If your patient has had a bowel movement, there will be an odor, but make no mention of this. The patient knows an odor is present after a bowel movement. He has just performed a normal bodily function, and it should be treated as such. Even if you say nothing regarding odors in the room, the patient will be watching your face for any signs of disgust or dislike. Be careful your expression does not register any negative opinions.

Assist with cleansing the genital and rectal areas now if your patient needs help. Disposable wipes are handy, and you can wear disposable gloves. Commercial sprays are available which help cleanse bowel movement from the skin. You may also use soap and water, always wiping in the direction of the rectum.

Some patients are too weak to lift their hips, and you will not be able to slide the bedpan underneath them. In this instance, have your patient turn onto his side. Then position the pan against the buttocks and thigh area, and assist the patient to turn back onto the pan. (Hold the bedpan securely in place with one hand while he turns back onto it.)

To remove your patient from the bedpan, hold the pan securely with one hand, while you use the other to help turn the patient off the pan. If your loved one is very weak or ill, you might need the assistance of another person to help place and remove the bedpan.

For males, the male urinal will be fine for passing urine, although some males cannot void in a sitting position. In such a case you may need to help your patient stand at the bedside. For the bed or chair confined patient who is confused or very weak, place the urinal for him. Ask him to spread his legs slightly and position the urinal in a slightly tilted downward angle between his legs. Then gently place his penis into the urinal. You can pad the urinal with a towel and leave it in place for a few minutes. Avoid putting undue pressure on the scrotum while placing the urinal.

If you are a female, a male family member can place the urinal for you. Most males will be able to place the urinal themselves, so you will probably only need to hand your patient the urinal and give him privacy.

Provide a washable cover for the bedpan or urinal (or use a disposable linen saver), and empty its contents promptly. Carry the bedpan or urinal to a commode to empty it, and then rinse with cold water. You may use a disinfectant solution to rinse the utensil. A commode brush swishes away any bowel movement that does not readily rinse from the bedpan.

Adding a small amount of both disinfectant and water to the pail of the bedside commode helps control odors. You can spray the utensil with spray disinfectant also. Spray your patient's room if odor is a problem. Small electric air fresheners used to clear cigar and cigarette smoke will help with odors, too.

When finished with toileting, always wash your own hands and your patient's hands. Have a special area to store the bedpan or urinal. Do not place it on the over-the-bed table or any other surface where food and bathing supplies are placed. Nor should you place it on the floor where it would pick up bacteria that could be transferred to your patient's bed.

▶ BED MAKING

Making an Unoccupied Bed

If your patient is able to get up, make the bed as you would make any unoccupied bed. However, you may wish to add a turning or lifting sheet and incontinence pads if needed. Changing bed linens daily is unnecessary, but do change sheets when they are soiled and completely change all linens at least weekly.

When removing soiled linens from the bed, avoid shaking them in the air. Shaking scatters any bacteria on the soiled sheets into your patient's sickroom. Merely loosen all sheet corners, place them to the center of the bed, and then carry the sheets to the laundry. Clean the mattress with a disinfectant, but do not soak the mattress covering. Wring the cloth out well. The headboard, footboard, and bed frame should also be washed weekly, a job that will only take a few minutes.

Make square hospital corners with your sheets if you know how, but do not be concerned if you can not make them. Just use fitted sheets for the bottom sheets and tuck the top sheets as you usually do on your own bed.

Making an Occupied Bed

Although it seems impossible to make a bed with your patient lying in it, with practice you will master this procedure. It is only necessary to make an occupied bed if your patient cannot be gotten out of bed. Work in an orderly fashion. Collect all linens and have them nearby. Linens should be folded lengthwise because this will form a crease down the center of the sheet, making centering the sheet easier.

To begin, raise the side rail and turn your patient to that side of the bed which is away from you. The patient's back will be toward you, and you will change the side of the bed near you first. Make sure your patient is comfortable. Position a pillow beneath the head. (It may be necessary to turn the pillow lengthwise to give yourself more working area.)

Working on the opposite side of the bed from your patient, loosen the bottom sheet and then the other linens, and tuck them to the center of the bed as close to your patient's body as possible. Using the center crease as a guideline, position the clean sheets on the bed, and fold back and tuck near to your patient the portions of the sheets that are to go to the other side of the bed. Position incontinence pads if needed, again folding in half and tucking the folded portion next to your patient.

The half of the bed near you should now contain all bottom sheets. You are ready to turn your patient to the clean side of the bed. Raise that side rail and assist the patient to roll over the folded linen. Depending on the linens needed, there may be a large mound of linens to roll over. Warn the patient about this. You can say, "I want you to come over to my side of the bed now. You'll feel a big hump when you turn." (See Figure 3.)

For safety, always be certain the rail is raised on the side of the bed which the patient is turned toward. If you have to leave the bedside, even for a few seconds, be certain both side rails are raised.

Now, going to the other side of the bed, lower the side rail and remove the soiled linens. The clean linens are ready to be tucked into place. Your patient can then be turned onto his back and the top linens

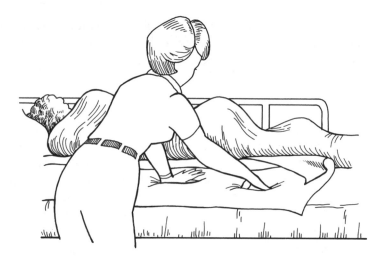

Figure 3. Making an occupied bed. The caregiver has completed the near side of the bed and is ready to turn the patient onto that side, so she can complete the other.

applied. Do not tuck the top sheets too tightly over the toes. This may cause discomfort, and bedsores have been known to develop on the tips of toes due to the top sheets being applied too tightly. Change the pillow cases, and the occupied bed has now been completely changed.

While making your patient's occupied bed, you changed all the bottom sheets on one side of the bed before changing the other side of the bed. Then you applied the top sheets. This procedure of bed making is orderly, and you are not tiring yourself by walking from one side of the bed to the other. Use this same procedure when making an unoccupied bed; change one entire side of the bed, including top sheets, before moving to the other side of the bed to complete the bed making.

Tending to your patient's personal care may seem complicated, but with practice you will perform these procedures in a short amount of time. Do not strive for perfection when first attempting to give a bed bath or to make an occupied bed. Adapt the procedure to your specific patient, depending on his condition and needs. Always practice rules of good safety and work with a gentle touch. The ill person who can perform personal care, either completely or partially, may be very slow, and you could probably do it in half the time, but have patience and allow the patient to do as much for himself as possible.

CHAPTER 4

SPECIAL SKIN CARE

▶ INSPECTING THE SKIN

You may not realize it, but you have now become an inspector and a detective. While bathing your patient, you should constantly observe the skin. Watch for irritation, rashes, and excessive dryness, and also note the color and temperature of the skin.

Good skin care is essential to all, but it is especially important to elderly patients because their skin is more delicate, with wrinkles, sagging, thinning, and a general loss of elasticity. The skin may have blotchy, spotty areas of pigmentation, brown spots, age spots, bumpy raised scales resembling warts, and dry flaking.

Consult your physician if you notice bleeding or a change in size or color of any mole or other suspicious sore. The greatest skin care problem to any ill person, regardless of age, however, is bedsores.

▶ BEDSORES

Bedsores, also called pressure sores or decubitus ulcers, occur as a result of skin breakdown. This happens when an area of skin tissue does not get proper blood circulation or is subjected to pressure. A bedsore can form anywhere on the body, but bony areas where the bone is prominent under the skin are more prone to breakdown. These areas include the elbows, heels, sacrum (base of the spine), shoulder blades, ankles, and sides of the hips. Bedsores can also occur where two areas of skin are in constant contact, such as the abdominal apron or beneath the breasts. Bedsores on the outer ear and back of the head are not uncommon to the bed patient. The wheelchair patient may develop bedsores on the lower buttocks or behind the knees. (See Figure 1.)

Some patients are more prone to bedsores than others. If your patient is up and about a good deal of the time, he probably will not develop a bedsore, but the patient who is in bed a good deal of time or sitting in a wheelchair may develop a bedsore quickly. Elderly persons with poor circulation are prone to bedsores. Other factors which contribute to bedsores are poor skin care, failure to change the body

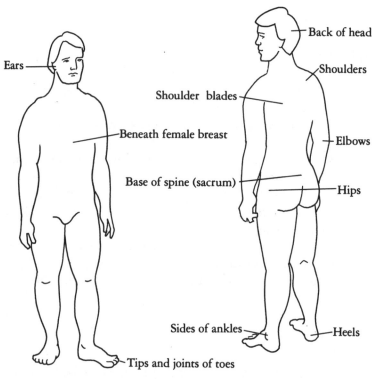

Figure 1. Common locations of bedsores.

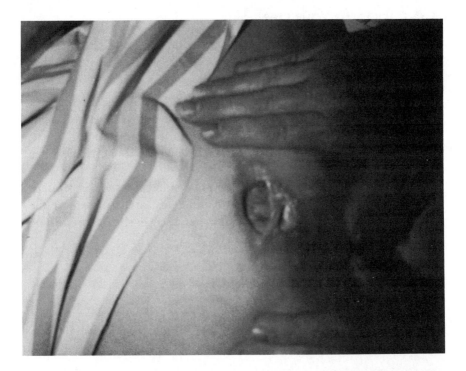

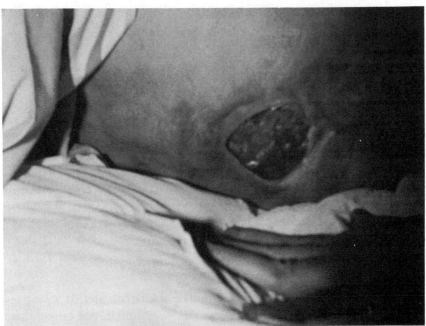

Figure 2. This patient has two bedsores. In the top figure, the bedsore is located on the hip. In the bottom figure, it is located at the sacrum.

position frequently, poor nutrition and dehydration, poor control of urine and bowel movements, and loss of sensation (e.g., a paralyzed person).

Prevention is the best treatment for a bedsore. A slight redness of tissue, especially at the bony areas, is the first sign of a bedsore. Left untreated, this redness could develop into a large, painful, open, draining sore to a depth that eventually involves bone tissue. (See Figure 2.)

Even though you have been giving good skin care, such as massaging with lotion, applying powder to skin folds, and so forth, at the first signs of skin redness or tenderness, special skin care will be needed to prevent further skin damage.

Special Skin Care Measures

Special skin care measures can help with circulation, comfort, and healthy skin. At the first sign of skin irritation, take the following measures.

1. Change your patient's position frequently. A healthy person shifts positions every few minutes, but your patient may not be able to do this. Turn or change your patient's body position every hour or two depending on his condition. Use a turning sheet or lift sheet to prevent scraping your patient over the bed because this will cause even more skin irritation.

2. To increase circulation to a reddened area, massage gently AROUND the area, but not directly over the reddened area as this may cause more damage to already damaged tissue. Do not use plastic on damaged skin. Plastic, such as a linen saver, collects moisture and does not allow air to circulate.

3. Apply lotion to your patient's skin to help decrease friction.

4. Keep the bed sheets free of wrinkles.

5. Provide a balanced diet to promote healing.

6. Control diarrhea and urinary incontinence to prevent further skin breakdown.

7. Provide mild exercise to stimulate the circulation. If your patient is unable to perform exercises for himself, you can do this for him. (For further discussion see Chapter 7.)

In addition, special products are available to aid in healing and to help prevent bedsores.

Water Mattress. A water mattress is placed on the bed and then filled with water and is similar to a water bed. This mattress exerts less pressure on the skin than a standard bed mattress.

Egg Crate Mattress. An egg crate mattress is a thin foam mattress about two inches thick, resembling an egg crate with "hills and valleys." It is placed on top of a regular mattress. Like the water mattress it also exerts less pressure on the skin; furthermore, its design allows air to circulate beneath the patient.

Alternating Air Mattress. An alternating air mattress is a thin mattress placed on top of a regular mattress. It consists of tubular coils which are filled with air. A small, quiet motor beneath the bed constantly changes the air in the coils; thus some coils are inflated while others are deflated, alternating the pressure on the skin.

Sheepskin Pads, Heel and Elbow Protectors. Pads and protectors reduce friction to a specific area. Soft and fluffy sheepskin pads are placed beneath the patient from the mid-back to the mid-thigh area. Heel and elbow protectors are designed to specifically fit these areas and are made of sheepskin or a layer of foam. The heels and elbows of those who have to spend a good deal of time in bed are subjected to much pressure. For example, bed patients use their elbows to help raise themselves to a sitting position, and therefore stress is placed on this delicate, bony area.

Gel Floatation Pads. Gel floatation pads are filled with a special gel substance. They work much like a water mattress and are especially helpful to a wheelchair patient.

In order to achieve the greatest benefit from these protection devices, place only the minimum amount of linen over them. For instance, if you use an alternating air mattress on your patient's bed, do not apply three or four layers of linens between the alternating air mattress and your patient as that will reduce the benefit. Use only one sheet beneath your patient when using an alternating air mattress if possible.

Over-the-Bed Cradles and Foot Cradles. Over-the-bed cradles and foot cradles are metal or wooden frames which are used over the bed to keep the top sheets from irritating skin while still providing warmth. A foot cradle is useful if your patient's toes are irritated from the top bed sheets. Over-the-bed cradles are frequently used for burned patients who cannot tolerate the weight of a sheet on their injured skin.

Donuts. Donuts are sheets of foam about an inch thick which are cut into the shape of a donut and placed around a bedsore. They allow air to circulate to the sore while protecting the skin surrounding the sore and redistributing body pressure.

Positioning

Proper positioning of your bed patient promotes comfort and helps prevent bedsores and muscle contractures. A muscle contracture is a shortening of a muscle which causes deformity and loss of use of that muscle. Such a contracture usually occurs in the arms, hands, legs, and feet.

A condition known as foot drop can also occur when a patient is confined to bed a great deal of the time. Without support to the feet, the foot gradually begins to droop downward, and after a time the muscles and ligaments in the top of the foot stretch and become accustomed to the drooping position. It takes months of exercise to return these muscles to their original positions, and the patient with severe foot drop will be unable to walk due to the deformity of the foot. A footboard can be used to support the feet of the bed-confined patient to prevent foot drop. Your physical therapist can suggest other devices for this problem. (See Figure 3a.)

Pillows and folded towels can be used to position your patient. When repositioning your patient in bed, keep the body in a natural position to prevent strain and discomfort. It is not always necessary to completely turn your patient from side to side or side to back to make a change in position. If your patient is lying on his side, you can reposition the pillows and turn him about 15 degrees toward the back position. Although you have not drastically changed his position, you have still redistributed weight and pressure on his body.

Use pillows, regular bed pillows and small, fairly flat toss pillows, to support the patient when you change positions and to help keep bony areas from rubbing on the bed or against each other. If you place your patient in the side position or partially on his side, place a bed pillow at the back and hips to provide comfort for your patient and to help hold him in that position. Lying in the side position, one knee is usually placed on top of the other causing skin irritation and breakdown. To prevent this, double a bath towel or fold a flannel sheet and place it between the knees. Whatever you use does not need to be thick to provide protection. (See Figure 3b.)

To protect the heels while your patient is lying in the back position, raise them slightly off the bed by placing a folded bath towel at the lower leg and ankle area. The heels need to be propped only an inch or

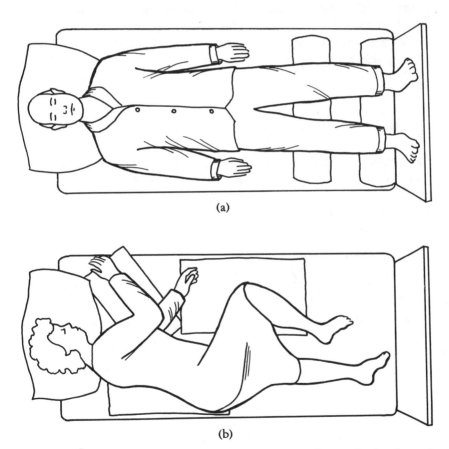

(a)

(b)

Figures 3. Common bed positions. Figure 3a shows the back position using a footboard. Figure 3b shows the side position.

two from the bed mattress. Use heel protectors along with raising your patient's heels from the bed to assure even greater protection. With lower legs slightly elevated to keep heels from rubbing against the mattress, your patient will also need some support beneath the knees because they will also be slightly elevated. Use a folded towel or a fairly flat toss pillow beneath the knees.

The patient who keeps his fists tightly clinched will need a soft sponge ball placed in his palms to prevent deformity of the hand and fingers. This is commonly seen in the paralyzed hand of a stroke patient.

If your patient is up and about and only lies in the bed for an afternoon nap and at nighttime, he probably changes positions frequently, and these measures will not be needed. However, even though he changes position often, his skin may be frail and susceptible to irritation. An egg crate mattress on the bed would be of benefit and stop any skin problems before they have a chance to start.

▶ OTHER SKIN PROBLEMS

The elderly person's sensation to temperature, pain, and touch are dulled. It is not uncommon for an aged person to be cut, burned, or bruised without noticing. Skin tears are common in the person with thin, paperlike skin.

Caring for Wounds

A deep, gaping, or profusely bleeding wound will require immediate care by a physician. Apply direct pressure to a bleeding wound, using a clean washcloth or dish towel until you reach medical help.

If the wound is small (e.g., a small cut or scrape), you can probably care for it yourself. Gently cleanse the wound with soap and water and pat dry. Apply an antiseptic or antibiotic ointment available at any drugstore.

To apply an ointment properly, do not use bare fingers. You may wear a disposable glove to apply the ointment, and once you touch the wound with your covered finger, do not return that finger to the container as this would spread bacteria from the wound into the container of ointment. Cotton-tipped applicators can be used instead of the finger. Use a clean applicator each time you return to the container for more ointment. Sterile, individually wrapped tongue depressors are available at the pharmacy if the wound is large and you need to apply a greater amount of ointment.

After the ointment has been applied, cover the wound with a gauze dressing and secure it with adhesive tape. A special adhesive tape resembling paper works well on delicate skin because it is porous and allows air to circulate beneath the tape. If your patient's skin is very thin or sensitive, avoid placing adhesive tape directly onto the skin. Instead, secure the dressing by wrapping rolled gauze around the affected area, and then place the tape over the gauze. (Of course, this method of wrapping can only be used on areas that allow circular wrapping such as the arms, legs, and forehead.) Gauze dressings impregnated with white petroleum jelly are helpful if the wound sticks to the dressing, which is common with skin tears.

For a small burn, immediate care includes the application of an ice pack or a cold, wet cloth to reduce the stinging sensation. Later you may apply an antiseptic or antibiotic ointment and dressing. If the burn is large or deep, produces blisters, is painful, or your patient has a fever, a physician should be consulted immediately. Change all dressings at least daily and inspect the wound for signs of infection, such as increased redness, swelling, pain, or drainage.

Itching

Itching is a common problem of many adults, and it is usually caused by dry skin. Itching could also be a sign of a drug reaction, allergies, an illness, or a skin disorder, so consult your physician if your patient's itching is severe. Itching that disturbs sleep should also be brought to the attention of a physician. Rectal itching is common in both the male and female elderly patient. Female vaginal itching is also common in the elderly patient. Your physician can treat these problems.

Following are some hints for controlling itching.

1. Keep your patient's fingernails short and encourage him to avoid scratching or rubbing the itchy area.
2. Your patient should wear loose, comfortable clothing.
3. If your patient is permitted tub baths, use as little soap as possible and rinse and dry his body well. Cornstarch or oatmeal can be added to the bath water to help ease itching.

4. Apply lotions, baby oil, or special ointments and creams available at the drugstore.

5. If itching persists, consult your physician.

▶ SPECIAL FOOT CARE

A decrease in the skin sensation and poor blood circulation of the elderly patient makes foot care especially important. If ignored, the slightest nick on the foot or toe of a person with poor circulation could lead to an infection and possibly eventual gangrene.

As the caregiver, you are constantly inspecting and observing your patient. Bathe and inspect the feet daily. Spread the toes and examine the area between the toes for cracks or signs of infection. Inspect the soles of the feet as well as the tops. Look for sores, cracks, irritations, swelling, discoloration, corns, and calluses. Examine the toes for signs of ingrown nails. Overlapping and webbed toes are a constant source of irritation and infection.

Proper Foot Care

The following procedures will help the caregiver administer proper foot care.

1. Inspect your patient's feet daily. The feet should be soaked in warm water at least weekly, and daily if your patient is a diabetic. A few minutes is long enough. Avoid the shriveled prune look.

2. Dry the feet thoroughly, especially between the toes.

3. Apply lotion or baby oil, but use powder between the toes and webbed spaces.

4. Foot powder may be applied if the feet perspire heavily.

5. Trim nails as needed by cutting straight across, and file the rough spots with an emery board. Nail trimming should be performed by a podiatrist (foot doctor) if your patient is a diabetic, has poor circulation, or if nails are very thick.

6. Exercise your patient's feet daily. (Range of motion exercises for the feet are described in Chapter 7.)

7. Your patient should wear properly fitting shoes.

8. Your patient should wear clean socks daily, preferably white cotton.

9. Your patient should avoid wearing garters or other restrictive bands about the legs.

10. Your patient should avoid sitting with knees crossed because this decreases blood circulation to the leg and foot.

11. Your patient should avoid walking barefoot.

12. Do not use iodine or other harsh antiseptics on your patient's feet.

13. Do not apply electrical heating pads or hot water bottles to the feet of an elderly person.

14. Apply bedsocks, extra thick stockings, or two pairs of stockings if your patient's feet tend to be cold.

Special Nail Care

Due to the aging process with a lessening of circulation to the extremities, most elderly persons have thick and brittle toenails. If your patient has very poor circulation, is a diabetic, has corns and calluses or very thick toenails, it is advisable to have a podiatrist care for his feet. Some podiatrists do make home calls for the patient who is confined to the bed or the home. If you have any doubt about caring for your patient's feet, consult a podiatrist before attempting to trim nails or treat corns or calluses.

CHAPTER 5

FOODS AND FLUIDS

▶ MEALTIME FOR THE PATIENT

Maintaining a well-balanced diet for the patient now residing with you may not be an easy task. Old age brings a decreased sense of taste and smell, chewing difficulties, and less physical activity, which requires fewer calories. Mealtime should be a social time for your patient. You may have chosen breakfast as a time to be with your family, but after the morning routine of bathing and personal hygiene is completed, take a coffee or juice break with your patient.

Your patient will enjoy meals more if he can be gotten out of bed, and even more so if he can walk or be taken by wheelchair to the table. Encourage your patient to eat with others. Mealtime is more pleasant if the meal is shared. If your patient is unable to get out of bed, carry your lunch to his room and share the mealtime.

Encourage your patient to invite friends for a morning or afternoon snack or to share a meal. This need not be complicated. A simple soup, sandwich, and salad will be fine for lunch.

If your patient has poor eating habits, do not expect to change these habits in a few days. The patient who has simply drunk a cup of coffee for breakfast for the last twenty years will not be anxious to eat a huge breakfast of toast, scrambled eggs, juice, and bacon. Start by offering only orange juice along with the coffee and gradually increase the amount of food. Breakfast is an important meal, and usually the person with a poor appetite feels hungrier and eats more for breakfast than at other meals.

Some patients may experience indigestion after consuming a large meal three times a day, and for them more frequent, smaller feedings are better. Some elderly patients will eat well one day and then only nibble the next.

▶ THE FOUR BASIC FOOD GROUPS

Knowing what foods provide the best nutritional value is important. Besides nutritional value, food should look attractive, be colorful, and provide a variety of textures (unless roughage is a problem). Foods are classified into four basic groups. Use these groups as a guideline for planning your patient's meals (see Figure 1).

A Selection of Foods from the Four Basic Food Groups

I Milk Group	II Vegetable and Fruit Group	III Meat Group	IV Bread and Cereal Group
Milk	Apples	Ham	Cereal
Dried Milk	Oranges	Chicken	Bread
Skimmed Milk	Bananas	Turkey	Rice
Ice Cream	Grapes	Beef	Flour
Evaporated Milk	Carrots	Fish	Oatmeal
Swiss Cheese	Asparagus	Fish Sticks	Crackers
Creamed Chese	Broccoli	Oysters	Bisquits
Cottage Cheese	Lettuce	Dried Peas	Spaghetti
Yogurt	Green Peppers	Dried Beans	
	Prune Juice	Peanut Butter	
	Grapefruit Juice		

Figure 1. The four basic food groups.

The Milk Group

Choose at least two servings daily from the milk group. This should include eight ounces of whole, skimmed, dried, or evaporated milk or buttermilk. You may also choose milk products, such as 1 1/2 ounces of cheese, 1 1/3 cups of cottage cheese, 1 2/3 cups of ice cream, or 1 cup of yogurt. If your patient does not like milk, use it in puddings, creamed soups, and in cooking.

The Vegetable and Fruit Group

Choose at least four servings daily from the vegetable and fruit group. Serve 1/2 cup of fruit juice, such as orange, grapefruit, or tomato juice daily, and also serve fresh fruits, such as apples, bananas, grapefruits, or cantaloupe. Your menu should include 1/2 cup of vegetables, such as broccoli, potatoes, carrots, pumpkin, tomatoes, and cabbage. Dark green and yellow vegetables are also a good source of vitamin A and should be served daily. Provide a good source of vitamin C every day. Foods high in vitamin C include citrus fruits or juices, broccoli, brussels sprouts, cantaloupe, and strawberries.

The Meat Group

Choose at least two servings daily from the meat group. This should include at least two to three ounces of lean meat, poultry, or fish. Meat provides protein which is needed for cell building in the body. One egg or 1/2 cup cooked dried beans or peas also provides protein. Peanut butter is another good source of protein.

The Bread and Cereal Group

Choose at least four servings daily from the bread and cereal group. Serve one slice of whole grain or bread made from enriched flour or a similar baked good daily. You may also choose one ounce of ready-to-eat cereal, 1/2 cup cooked cereal, spaghetti, noodles, macaroni, or rice. Two graham crackers or five saltines can replace a slice of bread if preferred.

▶ A POOR APPETITE

You will have no problem providing a balanced diet for the person who eats well, but if your patient has a poor appetite, mealtime will pose many problems. There are numerous causes for a loss of appetite, and if possible, these causes should be eliminated. Some causes of a poor appetite in the elderly patient, however, cannot be eliminated, such as a decreased sense of smell and taste. A decrease in the amount of saliva in the mouth is also common for a person in the late 70s or older and can cause a poor appetite.

On the other hand, some causes of a poor appetite can be eliminated.

1. Tooth decay and gum disease make the chewing of food not only painful, but also embarrassing. Consult your dentist for advice.

2. Poorly fitted dentures also make chewing food difficult and embarrassing. Again, consult your dentist. The dentures will need to be replaced or relined. Encourage your patient to wear the dentures. He will feel better knowing he looks attractive, and it will eliminate serving "baby food" meals.

3. Medications sometimes cause a loss of appetite and/or nausea. Ask your physician for assistance if this is a problem.

4. Emotional problems can cause a poor appetite. Depression is common in the elderly. A sense of loss is usually the cause of depression. This loss may involve the loss of a loved one, such as a spouse with whom the patient shared many years. Loss of a sense of self-worth may come about because the elderly or chronically ill person is no longer able to work.

   The person who is ill could have a poor body image, especially if he is no longer able to move about the way he once could. Consult your physician if your patient has any of these problems.

5. Poor digestion and indigestion also contribute to a poor appetite. Hiatal hernia, a condition in which part of the stomach slides up along the esophagus and in turn produces inflammation of the lower esophagus, is common in the elderly. This condition causes gas and heartburn after eating. Choose foods that are soft and easy to digest, such as creamed soups,

puddings, and cream of wheat. Avoid highly spiced foods. Antacids will help relieve the gas and heartburn, and eating smaller meals more frequently will also help. Have your patient sit in an erect position while eating, and he should not lie down directly after eating. Remaining in a sitting position will help food pass through the hernia area.

Besides being prone to hiatal hernias, the elderly also have a decrease in the amount of secretion of enzymes and bile needed for digestion which slows down the digestion process.

6. Constipation is a common problem of the elderly and chronically ill which also causes a loss of appetite. (Constipation is discussed in Chapter 6.)

7. The financial circumstances of retirement sometimes cause an older person to eat poorly. For some retired persons decreased income is a very real problem, and they must reduce the amount of money spent on food.

Supplemental Feedings and Snacks

Supplemental feedings and snacks should be provided for the patient with a poor appetite. Avoid serving snacks containing high amounts of sugar and no nutritive value (e.g., candies and cakes). The poor eater needs foods high in protein and calcium. Cheese-flavored crackers with peanut butter, milk shakes, cheese and saltines, ice cream, puddings, custards, and raisins are recommended.

Carnation® Instant Breakfast[1] drink is a good between-meal drink that is high in protein, comes in a variety of flavors, and can be served hot or cold. Ask your doctor about using this drink. It is especially important to consult your physician if your patient is a diabetic because that patient's diet will have to be closely monitored. A No Sugar Added Carnation® Instant Breakfast is now available which is sweetened with NutraSweet®. Dietitians have successfully included this variety in diabetic diets. Carnation® Instant Breakfast drinks are inexpensive and can be purchased at a local supermarket.

Ensure® Liquid Nutrition[2] is a good-tasting, all-purpose liquid food providing complete, balanced nutritional support. Ensure® can be used as a diet supplement or total feeding and is available in a variety of flavors, which can be purchased or ordered from a local pharmacy. Consult your physician before using this product, especially if your patient is a diabetic.

Offer snacks frequently to the poor eater without being overzealous about coaxing the patient to eat more. Have snacks readily available, but be certain your patient is not eating too many snack foods and ruining his appetite for mealtimes.

Encourage your patient to smell the food. Actually being able to smell food helps to stimulate the appetite. (This is why you do not feel like eating when you have a cold that hinders your sense of smell.)

If your patient has a poor appetite, offer nutritious drinks such as milk shakes and eggnog. Use your imagination to create drinks using a variety of fruits and flavorings. Following are the recipes for some drinks you can make.

◆ *Chocolate Frost Shake* ◆

1 tbsp. cocoa
1 tbsp. sugar
1 cup milk
1 scoop vanilla ice cream

Add sugar, cocoa, and small amount of the milk to a blender and blend well. Add remaining milk and ice cream and blend. For variations try $1/2$ tsp. instant coffee for a mocha flavor. Add peppermint extract to taste for a minty chocolate flavor.

◆ *Pineapple Milk Shake* ◆

Puree in blender
1 cup pineapple juice
Add
$1/4$ cup cream of coconut
1 cup milk
1 cup vanilla ice cream
Blend together and serve over crushed ice.

◆ *Orange Drink* ◆

2 tbsp. frozen orange juice concentrate
4 ice cubes crushed

$^1/_2$ cup milk
Add sugar to taste.
Mix together in a blender and serve.

Weighing the Patient

Weighing your patient regularly is your best gauge to determine weight loss or gain. The very thin person probably will not want to be reminded of his thinness by being weighed daily, but weigh him at least weekly, preferably at the same time of the day (before breakfast), wearing the same amount of clothing. Keep a record of the patient's weight in your notebook.

Persons who are prone to retaining fluid, such as in swelling of the feet (pedal edema), should be weighed daily, preferably in the morning. Keep an accurate weight record in your notebook.

Hints To Promote a Good Appetite

In addition to the suggestions already made, the caregiver may find the following list helpful in promoting a good appetite.

1. Offer your patient the use of the toilet prior to meals.
2. Offer mouth care prior to eating, if indicated.
3. Have your patient wash his hands before eating.
4. Your patient should be free of pain and sitting in a comfortable position to eat.
5. Provide napkins. If your patient is an untidy eater, use a bib. A hand towel with ties to secure it about the neck works well. Refrain from using infant bibs, and refrain from calling it a "bib." Saying "Here is your napkin," as you fasten it around the neck is better.
6. Encourage the patient to feed himself if at all possible. Avoid scolding or ridiculing if he does happen to spill food or drink.
7. Mealtime should be a social time. Avoid loud noise, music, and so forth. This is not the time for a family squabble.
8. Your patient should chew food slowly. Avoid rushing meals.
9. Cut meats and vegetables into small bite-size pieces.
10. Serve hot foods hot, but test them first to avoid burning.
11. Offer your patient the use of the toilet after meals.

Special eating utensils are available for the patient who has difficulty feeding himself. Thick foam pads are available for handles of silverware for the patient with arthritis who has difficulty gripping the utensil. Cups which are not easily tipped over are available also.

If your patient chokes easily or has difficulty chewing, you may wish to puree some foods, such as meats and certain vegetables, in a blender. Use small amounts of water, broth, or sauce to help liquify food. The general rule is: Do not puree if ground foods will do; do not grind if diced will do.

▶ Special Diets

Low Salt and No Added Salt Diet

The low salt and no added salt diet may also be called a low sodium or a sodium restricted diet. The doctor will prescibe the diet, depending on the condition of your patient, and tell you exactly how much salt is permitted. Salt holds fluid in the body tissues; therefore, it is especially important to avoid salt if your patient retains fluid or has a heart problem or high blood pressure.

A *No Added Salt Diet* means that you are not to use the salt shaker at the table. It also means you are to avoid foods that are very high in salt content.

A *Low Salt Diet* is restricted to about 2000 mg (milligrams) or 2 grams of salt daily. Learn to be a label reader to determine the salt content of foods.

Foods to be avoided on low sodium diets include:

1. Smoked, processed, or cured meats, such as ham, bacon, corned beef, lunch meats, hot dogs, and sausage
2. Bouillon cubes and meat sauces
3. Salted snacks, such as potato chips, pretzels, and popcorn
4. Relishes, olives, Worcestershire sauce, and pickles
5. Baked goods prepared with baking soda or baking powder
6. Canned meats and canned vegetables
7. Sauerkraut in any form
8. Anchovies, sardines, canned tuna, and salmon

9. Cheese and peanut butter unless specially prepared without salt

10. Products listing such as disodium phosphate, monosodium glutamate, sodium benzoate or sodium on the label

11. Medications high in sodium such as some stomach alkalizers and laxatives. (Consult a pharmacist regarding the salt content of these products.)

Processed, smoked, cured, and canned foods are highest in salt. Fresh or frozen fruits and vegetables are low. Ask your doctor about using salt substitutes. You can also improve the flavor of foods by using other spices, but not those containing salt, such as celery salt, onion salt, or garlic salt. Lemon juice can be used to improve the flavor of fish.

Mrs. Dash®[3] is a commercially prepared mixture of natural herbs and spices which contains no sodium. It adds flavor and is permitted on low salt diets.

For help with a low salt diet a list of the sodium content of some foods is provided. Following this list is a sample low sodium menu for breakfast, lunch, and dinner, using the four basic food groups.

Sodium Content of Some Foods *

Food	Amount of sodium in mg
Bacon, 1 strip	71
Canned corned beef, 3 slices	803
Cured ham, $1/4$ lb.	518
Sausage, 3 $1/2$ oz.	740
Frankfurter, $1/8$ lb.	550
Canned salmon, 3 $1/2$ oz.	387
Canned tuna in oil, 3 $1/2$ oz.	800
Canned tuna in water, 3 $1/2$ oz.	41
Green olives, 2 medium	312
Regular butter, 1 pat	99
Unsalted butter, 1 pat	1
Vanilla ice cream, 1 cup	82
Noodles, 1 cup	3

Source: Pennington, J.A.T., and H.N. Church, *Food Values of Portions Commonly Used.* 14th edition. Philadelphia: J.B. Lippincott, 1980.

White bread, 1 slice	117
Orange juice, 8 oz.	3
Banana, 1	1
Lima Beans, fresh, $5/8$ cup	1
Lima Beans, canned, $1/2$ cup	271
Lima Beans, frozen, $5/8$ cup	129
Sauerkraut, $2/3$ cup	747

Low Sodium Menu

Breakfast
Grapefruit juice
Hot oatmeal
French toast with syrup
Coffee, tea, or milk

Lunch
Low salt homemade minestrone soup
Baked veal pattie on roll
Buttered peas
Blueberry tart
Coffee, milk, or tea

Dinner
Tossed salad
Beef tips, mushrooms in a low salt brown sauce
Served over noodles
Baby carrots
Ice cream or pudding
Coffee, milk, or tea

Low salt snacks as desired
No salt at the table

High Fiber Diet

Food fiber, also known as roughage, is the part of plant food which is not broken down chemically by the digestion process. Fiber affects the consistency and bulk of the stool (bowel movement) and the speed with which it passes through the intestines. Fiber holds water. If your patient consumes foods high in fiber on a daily basis, he will notice bowel movements that tend to be bulkier and softer and pass more quickly and easily through the intestines.

Fiber relieves straining at bowel movements, along with the buildup of pressure resulting from straining. Physicians usually recommend a high fiber diet for such conditions as constipation, irritable bowel syndrome, diverticulosis, and hemorrhoids.

All fruits and vegetables contain fiber. Your patient should eat them raw or dried, including the skins. Choose cereals containing bran, wheat flakes or shredded wheat, granola, and oats. Choose breads made from whole wheat, cracked wheat, rye, or raisins. Special "high fiber" breads are available. Pastas (spaghetti, noodles, etc.) are not a good source of fiber if made from refined flour. Other sources of high fiber include raisin bran, sunflower seeds, sesame seeds, nuts, peanut butter, whole grain muffins, and bran muffins.

Low Fiber or Low Residue Diet

In certain conditions your physician may advise you to decrease the amount of fiber or residue in your patient's diet. Choose strained fruit juices, vegetables and fruits prepared without skins or seeds, and refined breads and flour products. Milk is considered a medium residue food. If a low residue diet is prescribed, milk and milk products are usually limited to two cups a day.

Bland Diet

A bland diet may be recommended for those suffering with stomach ulcers or other stomach conditions. Bland diet means exactly that— bland foods. Avoid any foods which cause distress, such as raw vegetables, beans, cabbage, cucumbers, and any food that causes gas. Fruits should be served without seeds or skins. Your patient should avoid spices and highly seasoned foods, such as sausages and frankfurters. Avoid high fiber foods, such as bran cereals and nuts. Fried foods may cause distress and should be avoided along with highly flavored seasonings, such as chili sauce and barbecue sauce. Coffee, tea, alcohol, and colas may also cause distress. Today, most bland diets are very liberal. Physicians usually instruct their patients to avoid all foods which cause distress.

Low Cholesterol Diet

Much has been said about the link between the consumption of fatty foods containing high levels of cholesterol and heart disease and hardening of the arteries. Basically, fatty deposits containing cholesterol begin to line the inner arteries, and eventually these deposits harden and become tough. The arteries become narrow and lose their elasticity. This process, called atherosclerosis, interferes with circulation and is responsible for many heart attacks, heart disease, and strokes.

A diet of saturated fat (butter, coconut oil, and fat of meat) increases the amount of cholesterol in the blood. Polyunsaturated fats (corn oil, cottonseed oil, and safflower oil) lower the level of cholesterol in the blood. A diet high in fiber may also play a role in reducing cholesterol. Exercise, hereditary tendencies, and hormones also influence the amount of cholesterol in the blood.

Foods of plant origin contain no cholesterol. Fruits, vegetables, grains, cereals, nuts, and vegetable oils (except coconut oil and palm oil) are recommended for a low cholesterol diet.

Here are some general rules for a low cholesterol diet, followed by a sample menu which uses the four basic food groups.

1. Eat small portions of meat (six ounces per day) that contain less fat. Eat less beef, pork, lamb, and regular cheese. Instead, choose fish, poultry, and low fat cottage cheese.

2. Avoid whole milk and dairy products made from whole milk. Use skimmed or nonfat milk instead.

3. Your physician will limit the use of eggs. Usually two or three eggs per week are allowed. You may use egg substitutes.

4. Use polyunsaturated (unsaturated) oil for cooking and baking. Choose margarines which are polyunsaturated.

Low Cholesterol Menu

Breakfast
Grapefruit half
Bran flakes
Scrambled eggs made from egg substitute
Coffee, tea, or milk

Lunch

Tossed Salad
Spaghetti with meat sauce
Seasoned green beans
Sliced peaches
White bread
Coffee, tea, or milk

Dinner

Applesauce
Baked chicken thighs
Baked potato
Spinach with vinegar
Gingerbread with lemon sauce
Whole wheat bread
Coffee, tea, or milk

No butter—Use polyunsaturated margarine

Caffeine. Persons with heart conditions also may be told to decrease the amount of caffeine they consume. There is a wide difference in the caffeine content of beverages, depending on the brand and method of preparing or brewing. Other beverages besides coffee contain caffeine, for example, tea, cocoa, and cola drinks. If your patient has a heart condition, the physician will probably recommend that you serve decaffeinated coffee and tea and avoid other drinks high in caffeine. The person who sleeps poorly or complains of being nervous or "jittery" might also benefit by eliminating caffeine drinks.

High Protein Diet

A decrease in the amount of protein consumed is often seen in elderly and other chronically ill patients. However, protein is especially important during illness and also helps with wound healing following surgery. Protein is found in all meats, eggs, cheeses, and milk products. Peanut butter, dried peas, and dried beans are also good sources of protein.

On the other hand, certain patients, for example, those with some types of kidney diseases, may need to restrict the amount of protein they consume. Your doctor or dietitian will help plan a diet which limits foods high in protein.

Weight Reduction Diet

Physicians often prescribe a diet with a specified number of calories for the overweight person. If your patient is on such a diet, it is important to follow the physician's orders exactly. See that your patient eats a well-balanced diet of foods from the four basic food groups daily. Under no circumstances resort to the use of fad diets or fasting to lose weight.

▶ FEEDING THE PATIENT

If your patient is unable to feed himself, you may have to do this for him. For most adults, this will be a very demeaning procedure. Although you are feeding your patient, try to have him in control of the meal. For example, ask what food he would like first, and then ask if you are giving it too fast or too slowly. Some like to vary their food while eating; others eat one food completely before eating the next. Never hurry your patient, and offer small amounts of food to prevent choking. A flexible straw may be helpful with liquids. A feeding cup, resembling a baby's training cup, may be useful for those who choke easily on liquids.

▶ MEALTIME FOR THE CAREGIVER

As the caregiver, you must also see to it that your own dietary needs are met daily. You need to eat well-balanced meals to be in the best physical condition possible to care for your patient. Do not take shortcuts by skipping your own lunch because you are too busy preparing lunch for your patient.

Unless the patient is on a very strict diet, you will be able to prepare the same meal for both of you. For example, if your patient is on a two gram sodium restricted diet, you can prepare egg salad sandwiches, low sodium canned soup, and fresh fruit for the two of you. You can add salt to the soup and egg salad to suit your own taste.

Hints for Better Nutrition

The following hints will be helpful for better nutrition for you, your patient, and your family.

1. Do not skip meals.
2. Cook vegetables in as little water as possible to prevent loss of vitamins.
3. Eat a variety of foods.
4. Be a label reader.
5. Eat slowly and chew food well.
6. Avoid large, heavy meals.
7. Plan several days' menus in advance before grocery shopping.

▶ FLUID INTAKE

An adult needs 1500 to 3000 cc (approximately 1 ½ to 3 quarts) of fluid (liquids) daily. This seems like a great amount until you consider that every food contains water. The person who perspires heavily will need a high intake of fluids, as will the one suffering with a fever. Encourage your patient to drink at least five to eight glasses of fluid daily, such as water, juices, milk, coffee, and so forth. A good fluid intake aids digestion as well as helping to relieve constipation.

Usually, if your patient is not getting enough fluids, he will be thirsty. The mouth and tongue will appear dry, lips will be dry and cracked, skin will be dry, and eyes may appear sunken. Urine that is very concentrated (having a dark amber color) is also a signal that your patient is not drinking enough fluids. Furthermore, a decrease in the amount of urine is a sign of decreased fluid intake, and dehydration along with electrolyte imbalance may occur.

Your physician may instruct you to "force fluids" to your patient. This means that you offer fluids frequently throughout the day to increase fluid intake. You will be instructed on exactly how many glasses or cups of fluid to give daily (see Figure 2).

The average adult voids, or urinates, about 1 ½ to 2 quarts of urine daily. The patient who is vomiting will lose fluids during vomiting, and diarrhea also causes fluid loss. The patient who has a fever or is

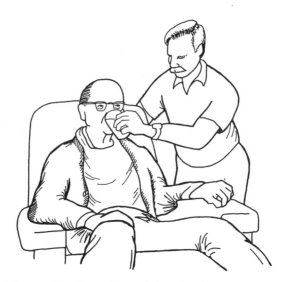

Figure 2.   Caregiver giving his father fluids.

perspiring may have dark urine because he is losing fluid in other ways besides urine (through the fever and perspiration).

The patient who is ill with a fever, vomiting, and diarrhea should be watched closely because dehydration and electrolyte imbalance can result.

If you are uncertain whether your patient is voiding a proper amount (called urinary output), measure the amount of urine voided. Have your patient void in the bedpan, urinal, or bedside commode, and using a disposable container which you have marked in 1/2 cup and cup increments, measure exactly how much is voided. Keep a record of the total amount voided in a 24-hour day. Your physician can use this to determine whether your patient is dehydrated. If severe dehydration does occur, your patient will probably be hospitalized and given intravenous (IV) fluids.

Electrolyte imbalance and dehydration usually occur together. You have no doubt heard your physician mention "electrolytes" or "electrolyte imbalance," but probably you are not quite sure what this means. Briefly, about two-thirds of the body fluid is found within the trillions of tiny cells in the body, and the other one-third is located outside or between the cells. Each cell contains tiny particles of chemical substances called electrolytes. Examples of these chemical substances are potassium, sodium, chloride, and sulfate. In order that the cells perform their duties properly, these electrolytes must be in the proper amount and balance. If the electrolytes are not in the proper balance, the cells will show signs of distress. Severe electrolyte imbalance will eventually lead to convulsions and coma.

You may wonder why your physician is particularly concerned about your patient's potassium level. If your patient is taking a diuretic medication to remove excess body fluid (such as in congestive heart failure) and this medication is known to deplete the body of potassium, your physician must be certain the potassium level of the blood does not drop below the normal range. Electrolytes can be monitored by a blood test.

In some illnesses it may be necessary for the physician to restrict or limit the amount of fluid taken in by your patient, and you will be instructed on exactly how many glasses of fluid to give daily.

CHAPTER 6

BOWEL AND BLADDER PROBLEMS

▶ CONSTIPATION

Your patient may suffer from one or more bowel or bladder problems while in your care. Constipation is a common bowel problem that may occur. No set amount of bowel movements or times between bowel movements defines constipation. Some persons normally have three bowel movements daily, while others have one bowel movement every three or four days. Constipation may be defined as difficult bowel movements with the passage of hard, dry stools. For some, constipation and the establishment of poor bowel habits may have started in early childhood. Constipation is aggravated by lack of activity, poor muscle tone, poor diet and fluid intake, laxative abuse, and straining at bowel movements. Emotional factors and some drugs also cause constipation. In addition, it may be caused by a medical problem such as diverticulitis or a bowel obstruction.

Symptoms of constipation include headache, a bloated feeling, loss of appetite and nausea, and the expelling of flatus (gas) both through the mouth by belching and through the rectum. The abdomen usually feels hard and is enlarged.

Laxative Use and Abuse

Some individuals, especially the elderly, feel they need to have a daily bowel movement, and to accomplish this, they may resort to giving themselves daily enemas or laxatives. Some feel they need a "good cleaning out" on a routine basis. They believe that bowel material will eventually "poison" the system, and a good cleaning out or "purging" will rid the body of poisons. Habitually resorting to the use of laxatives, enemas, and suppositories does nothing to establish normal bowel movements and only leads to further dependence on such aids. Laxatives, enemas, and suppositories are needed at times, and they can be used to help establish a regular bowel pattern. However, once regularity has been established, they should be discontinued.

Establishing Regularity

If your patient has constipation, taking some steps to promote regularity can be helpful. Following are five steps to help establish regularity.

1. Develop a regular time for bowel movements. It is thought that the greatest action of the intestines occurs following a meal, especially right after breakfast, so this is a good time to encourage your patient to move his bowels. This is also a good reason not to skip breakfast. A cup of hot liquid, such as coffee, tea, prune juice, or water sometimes helps.

2. Encourage your patient to eat foods high in fiber and roughage. Fiber helps to hold water and makes the stool bulkier and softer. Waste moves through the body quicker, and bowel movements become easier and more regular. Encourage your patient to eat raw or dried fruits and vegetables, fruit juices, bran and bran cereals, other high fiber cereals, and breads made from whole grains.

3. Your patient needs to drink adequate amounts of fluid, usually about eight glasses daily, as fiber needs fluid to help soften the stools.

4. Your physician can recommend stool softeners or natural grain products which add bulk and water to the bowel movement without the harsh effects of laxatives.

5. If at all possible, encourage your patient to establish a regular program of activity and mild exercise.

Administering a Fleet® Brand Ready To Use Disposable Enema [4]

There may be times, despite all efforts to avoid constipation, that it does occur. At these times, and if your patient is physically able to tolerate it, an enema may be necessary. Disposable soapsuds enemas are available at any pharmacy, but unless you have been properly trained in administering this enema (which involves introducing a large amount of water into the colon), you should not attempt it. NEVER ADMINISTER AN ENEMA IN THE PRESENCE OF ABDOMINAL PAIN, NAUSEA, OR VOMITING.

A Fleet® Enema is easy to administer and usually produces good results. It is available at any pharmacy, and the directions are included on the package. IF YOU ARE IN DOUBT ABOUT WHETHER YOU SHOULD ADMINISTER AN ENEMA, CONSULT YOUR PHYSICIAN OR HOME HEALTH NURSE. (Fleet® Enema should not be used in cases where congenital megacolon or congestive heart failure are known to exist. It should be used with caution in persons with impaired renal function or where a colostomy exists. Proper and safe use of the Fleet® Enema requires that the product be administered according to directions for use. Do not administer to children under two years of age. If after the enema solution is administered there is no return of liquid, contact a physician immediately as dehydration could occur. See full professional labeling for complete information on professional use.)

Warm the Fleet® Enema first by placing the bottle in a pan of warm water, being careful that the solution is warmed to body temperature but not hot. For best results your patient should lie on his left side with the right knee comfortably flexed. A knee-chest position is also recommended, but in this position the head is lowered, and most elderly patients will become dizzy. Do not attempt to give an enema while your patient is sitting on the commode or standing. Use a linen saver to protect the bed, and have a bedpan or bedside commode near. Wear gloves if you wish. Expose your patient's buttocks, but cover the lower legs with a sheet or bath blanket for protection from chills and to provide some degree of privacy.

Spread the buttocks and examine the anus (the rectal opening). If your patient has hemorrhoids, ask him to bear down slightly as this will help to open and identify the rectal opening. Remove the tip covering of the Fleet® Enema. The tip is already lubricated, but it should be checked prior to use, and more lubrication can be added if desired or necessary.

Have your patient take a few deep breaths while you gently and slowly insert the enema tip. If you meet with resistance, stop for a few seconds and then gently squeeze a small amount of the enema solution into the rectum; this will usually help advance the tip. If you continue to meet with resistance, STOP AND DISCONTINUE THE PROCEDURE. Continuation may result in abrasion or rupture of the colon.

Once the tip has been advanced, squeeze the bottle to administer its contents, although you will not be able to completely empty the bottle. If your patient complains of any pain, weakness, faintness, or dizziness during the procedure, stop and discontinue. Monitor your patient closely for any further side effects.

The Fleet® Enema is more effective if your patient is able to retain the solution for a few moments. You can place the patient on the bedpan or bedside commode immediately after giving the enema, but encourage him to hold the solution for a time before expelling it. Be sure your patient has a call bell and toilet tissue before you leave the room to allow privacy.

After your patient has expelled the enema, you may have to assist with cleansing of the perineal and rectal area. It is a good idea to place a linen saver under your patient's buttocks in the event that he expells more bowel movement or gas. Before emptying the bedpan or bedside commode, check the results of the enema. Observe the amount and color of stool, and look for unusual signs, such as blood, mucus, or pus. If your patient has hemorrhoids, a small amount of blood may be present occasionally, but if bleeding occurs frequently or if the amount is greater than just an occasional spotting, report it to your physician. Also report any mucus or pus if present.

Bowel movements should be brown in color. Black stools or stools resembling tar usually indicate bleeding in the stomach or high up in the intestines, and this should be reported immediately. Some medications, such as those containing iron (ferrous sulfate), produce black stools, and this should be of no concern. Pepto Bismol®[5], a commonly used over-the-counter upset stomach and diarrhea medication, can also cause a temporary darkening of the stools. Certain foods, such as beets, also can cause the stools to be red.

Fecal Impaction

A fecal impaction occurs when a hard, dry stool is present in the rectum and cannot be passed by a normal bowel movement. Usually your patient will complain of the symptoms of constipation, such as headache, bloating of the abdomen with belching of gas and passing gas by the rectum, and no bowel movement for several days.

Your patient will probably not be aware of the fact that he has an impaction of hard stool. Sometimes liquid bowel movement will actually seep around this blocked bowel movement, and your patient will have diarrhea. This condition can be very deceiving because when having diarrhea, it seems unlikely that a hard, fecal impaction could be present in colon or rectum. If you suspect your patient is impacted with hard stool, consult the physician or home health nurse. The nurse or physician will perform a digital rectal exam, and unless the impaction is high up in the colon, it can usually be felt.

The home health nurse will probably then administer a mineral oil enema (such as a Fleet® Brand Ready To Use Mineral Oil Enema) which softens the stool and acts as a lubricant to help pass the stool. This is usually followed by a soapsuds enema or a regular disposable enema to be certain the entire impaction is removed.

Steps to promote regularity, such as giving stool softeners, providing a high fiber diet, and increasing the amount of fluids consumed, should also be instituted to prevent the occurrence of further impactions.

Administering a Soapsuds Enema

ONLY administer a soapsuds enema to your patient if you have been properly trained in this procedure. The home health nurse can give assistance. As with all enemas, DO NOT ADMINISTER IN THE PRESENCE OF ABDOMINAL PAIN, NAUSEA OR VOMITING, OR IF APPENDICITIS IS SUSPECTED.

The procedure for administering a soapsuds enema is listed for review for those who have been trained in this procedure.

1. Assemble equipment and have your patient empty his bladder before proceeding. Wash your hands. You should wear disposable gloves during this procedure. Disposable soapsuds enema kits are available at any pharmacy, and a premeasured packet of castile soap is included. Use this equipment once, and throw

it away. Equipment includes: an enema bag, bed protector, bedpan or bedside commode, toilet tissue, and lubricant.

2. Prepare the enema bag. One quart of water is generally used for an adult, but if your patient is very frail or weak, he may not be able to retain this amount. The water should be 105° F. Use a bath thermometer to make certain the temperature is correct. Shut off the clamp on the enema tubing; then add soap and water to the bag. Open the clamp to allow the solution to run through the entire length of tubing, thus removing all the air in the tubing.

3. Protect the bed with disposable incontinence pads or use a rubber sheet covered with a flannel blanket. Have the bedside commode or bedpan near.

4. Position your patient in the same position as used for the disposable enema—on the left side with the right knee flexed. Drape your patient as much as possible with a flannel sheet to prevent chilling.

5. With a water-soluble lubricant, lubricate two inches of the rectal tip. Depending on the disposable kit, the tip may already be lubricated, but add more if you desire.

6. Raise the upper buttocks and expose the patient's rectum. Insert the tip of the rectal tube and ask your patient to take deep breaths as you gently rotate and continue to insert the rectal tube. If you have difficulty advancing the tubing, stop and discontinue the procedure. Insert the tip of the tubing three to four inches for an adult.

7. Unclamp tubing and slowly administer the enema solution. Hold the bag no more than 18 inches above your patient's rectum. Lower the height of the bag to lower the pressure and slow the rate of flow. Usually a soapsuds enema is more effective if it is given slowly. Instruct your patient to take slow, deep breaths at intervals while administering the solution. This will help him relax.

8. Observe your patient constantly while giving a soapsuds enema. If he complains of any pain, weakness, faintness, shortness of breath, or other ill effects or if the solution will not flow properly, STOP AND DISCONTINUE THE PROCEDURE.

9. You may clamp the tubing and stop administering the solution for a moment during this procedure if your patient has

difficulty retaining the solution. Some older adults will not be able to retain the solution.

10. Slowly and gently withdraw the rectal tube after the solution has been given. Leave some solution in the tubing as you withdraw, so air does not enter the rectum, or pinch off the tubing with your fingers before withdrawing.

11. Assist your patient with the bedpan or bedside commode; then provide privacy.

12. Check your patient frequently for any signs of faintness or dizziness. Dispose of equipment.

Hemorrhoids

Many persons suffer with hemorrhoids or piles. Hemorrhoids are dilated and enlarged veins present at the rectal area. These varicose veins can be internal (located inside the anal sphincter—the muscle at the end of the rectum) or external hemorrhoids which are located outside this muscle. External hemorrhoids can be seen by inspecting the rectal area. If your patient has external hemorrhoids, you may have noticed them while bathing the rectal area.

Hemorrhoids are caused by prolonged sitting or standing, pregnancy, chronic constipation, and straining at stools. Persons suffering with hemorrhoids tend to put off having bowel movements because the passage of stool, especially hard stool, is painful. However, delaying the bowel movement only causes more constipation and more straining. Hemorrhoids often cause bleeding. An occasional drop or two of blood on the toilet tissue or underwear is no cause for alarm, but if the bleeding is more severe and goes on for a long period of time, anemia could result. Hemorrhoids cause pain (especially with bowel movements) and an embarrassing itching.

Consult your physician for treatment. Many ointments and suppositories are available to ease the pain, itching, and swelling of hemorrhoids. A special bath called a sitz bath may soothe this condition.

A sitz bath is a regular tub bath in which the buttocks and hip areas are soaked in warm water. A rubber air ring is used to ease the pressure of sitting directly on the tub surface. The air ring is covered with a towel to make it even more comfortable. A commercially made sitz bath is available for the patient who cannot get into a bathtub. This plastic, basin-like container fits on the commode seat.

Warm compresses will also help soothe the rectal area, and it is important that your patient's constipation be remedied. Using stool softeners, eating a high fiber diet, and drinking plenty of fluids are recommended treatments. If the condition is severe, the hemorrhoids may be surgically removed.

▶ Diarrhea

Diarrhea is a condition in which the bowel movements are frequent and loose or liquid in consistency. An infection, an allergy to food or drink, a reaction to certain drugs, or emotional stress can cause diarrhea. This type of diarrhea usually only lasts for a short time. If you suspect that a medication is causing your patient's diarrhea, consult your physician. Withdrawal of a particular medication may be recommended. Intestinal diseases (such as colitis) cause diarrhea symptoms of longer duration, and you will need to discuss this with the physician.

The patient with diarrhea will pass an abnormal number of bowel movements which are either loose or liquid in consistency. Abdominal cramping or pain may occur, followed by a need to pass a bowel movement. If you have to inform your physician regarding the diarrhea, he will want to know exactly how many bowel movements your patient has passed and their consistency (e.g., watery, loose, semisoft, or mushy) and the amount of stool passed. You can estimate the amount of stool passed. For instance, it could be a few spoonfuls each time, half a cup, or a cup.

The physician will usually allow you to try an over-the-counter medication for diarrhea. Some diarrheas can be quickly eased by avoiding the food that is causing the disturbance. If emotional worries are causing the upset in the intestines, perhaps these worries can be overcome.

Diarrhea can become a very serious problem to the elderly, frail, or chronically ill person. It causes weakness, and there is a possibility of injury from a fall. If the diarrhea is left unchecked, it can lead to dehydration and electrolyte imbalance because of the large amount of fluids lost in the bowel movements. All persons suffering with diarrhea will need extra fluids to compensate for fluid loss. Any diarrhea that lasts more than one day should be reported to your physician. Consult your physician immediately if fever or pain occurs, or if the patient becomes dehydrated.

Your patient may be very upset and embarrassed if diarrhea occurs. This will be especially true if he cannot get to the toilet or bedpan in time or if you normally do not need to assist with cleansing, changing clothing, and so forth. Provide privacy and reassurance for your patient. Your attitude should be one of acceptance and understanding. Keep your patient and bed linens clean and dry. Handwashing is especially important after each toileting for you as well as your patient.

▶ POOR BOWEL CONTROL

The patient with poor bowel control poses a special problem. This person may be confused, suffering from diseases which cause poor perception of feeling the urge to pass a bowel movement, or may be extremely weak and debilitated. Whatever the cause, your loved one will probably be more upset and embarrassed about this lack of control than you are. No amount of ridicule or teasing on your part will solve this problem. Try to anticipate your patient's needs by placing him on the bedpan or bedside commode at certain times of the day, especially following meals. If this measure fails, however, you must accept the fact that he has poor control (incontinence) of bowel movement. Continue to provide a high fiber diet and encourage the intake of plenty of liquids.

Adult disposable diapers are available for such patients, and using linen savers on the bed will help with clean up. Specially made incontinence pants are also available. These are waterproof, and some have disposable liners. They can be worn under clothing without being detected.

Some factors you should consider in selecting an incontinence pad or diaper are:

1. Cost—Some incontinent patients will need the pad or diaper changed six to eight times daily or even more. This will become a costly item. Some suppliers provide discounts if diapers or pads are purchased by the case. Some drugstores also provide small discounts to senior citizens.

2. Protection—It would be useless to economize by purchasing a less expensive form of protection only to find that more diapers or pads are needed.

3. Worn under clothing—This is important if your patient is up and about and able to participate in activities outside the home.

4. Ease of use—Diapers and pads should be easy to apply and remove. If your patient has some bowel and bladder control, you need a product that can be quickly removed to facilitate getting to the commode on time.

5. Irritation—Refrain from using any protection that causes skin irritation.

6. Fit—Using a diaper that is too small or too large will only lead to skin irritation, inadequate protection, and discomfort.

Give scrupulous skin care to the patient incontinent of bowel movement. Wash the rectal and perineal area well after each bowel movement, rinse well, and then dry. If the skin shows any signs of irritation, apply a zinc oxide ointment, the same used for diaper rash in infants. Change the liner or diaper as soon as possible after soiling to prevent skin breakdown.

Your patient's rectal and perineal areas may become very inflammed and irritated. This occurs readily when diarrhea is present. Usually toilet tissue will cleanse bowel movement from the rectal area, but if this area is very inflammed, even using the softest toilet tissue will cause pain. The rectal area can become so irritated when a patient suffers with diarrhea that wiping the rectal area with toilet tissue actually causes bleeding. For these severe cases, using rolled cotton or cotton balls saturated with mineral oil to cleanse the area is not as traumatic to the inflammed, tender skin. Consult your physician. An ointment may be recommended to help heal the irritated tissue.

▶ URINE PROBLEMS

To be able to recognize urinary problems, you must first recognize normal urine. Normal urine is clear and straw colored. Urine of a lighter color is usually due to an abnormally high intake of fluids, or the kidney function is such that the kidneys are unable to concentrate the urine. A dark brown or amber color indicates a more concentrated urine, and encouraging more fluids is necessary. Orange urine indicates the presence of bile salts. Certain medications prescribed for a urinary infection, however, will also turn the urine orange, and the pharmacist will forewarn you. Blood in the urine may appear as bright red or it may be smoky or rusty in color. Milky, cloudy urine may indicate the presence of pus.

Normal urine has the same consistency as water. Urine that appears to be "grainy," thick, or has mucus or pus should be brought to the attention of your physician.

Normal urine is slightly aromatic. Acetone, which is sometimes present in the diabetic's urine, will produce a sweet, fruity smell. Strong, odorous urine may indicate an infection or the need to increase fluid intake.

The average adult produces about one and one-half quarts of urine daily.

Urinary Tract Infection

Inspecting the urine is simple if your patient voids in the bedpan or bedside commode, but if the patient uses the toilet, a problem may go undetected. Occasionally, and more often if you suspect problems, have your patient void in a container so that you may inspect the urine. Both men and women develop urinary tract infections, but the female is more prone to them because her urethra, the tube that carries the urine out from the bladder, is shorter. It is therefore easier for bacteria to enter her bladder.

The patient suffering with a urinary infection will usually show changes in the color, odor, and/or amount of urine produced. The color may be dark, white with the presence of mucus, or it may contain blood. It will probably be more odorous. Your patient may complain of pain across the bladder area, lower back, or flank (the sides of the back over the kidney area). This pain may be aggravated when passing urine. Complaints of frequency (the need to pass urine often) and burning while voiding are also noted. Your patient may be acutely ill with chills and fever and/or nausea and vomiting. If you suspect a urinary tract infection, consult your physician. A urine specimen will probably be needed. (For a discussion of this procedure see Chapter 12.)

Medication will be prescribed if your patient does have a urinary tract infection. Most of these medications are taken with a full glass of water, and usually the pharmacist will note this on the medication label.

Even though your patient has the need to urinate frequently and even though this causes burning, you still need to give plenty of fluids.

Keeping the urine slightly acidic helps prevent infections, and drinking cranberry juice is highly recommended to increase the acidity. Try to give about eight glasses of fluids a day, including water and fruit juices, unless otherwise ordered to restrict fluids. Give coffee and tea in moderation.

The need of proper cleansing of the perineal area from front to back is important. The female patient should also be instructed on the proper use of toilet tissue. When wiping with toilet tissue, she should wipe from the front to the back, again not distributing bacteria from the rectal area or vaginal area into the urinary opening. Some persons are also allergic to the color and scents used in toilet tissue, so plain white tissue is best for them.

A urinary tract infection is a very common condition to persons of any age. If your patient does develop this condition, provide the following care.

1. Give medications as ordered, usually with plenty of water.

2. Keep patient and bed linens clean and dry. The patient who has had good bladder control might lose proper control during a urinary tract infection.

3. Be observant for skin irritations. Cleanse the genital and rectal areas, thighs, and buttocks as needed with soap and water, rinsing, and then drying well. Bedsores are more likely to develop with poor urinary control.

4. Keep the bedpan, urinal, or bedside commode near. If your patient is able to use the toilet, help him to the toilet at regular intervals.

5. Give fluids as ordered.

6. Because the urine may have a stronger odor during a urinary tract infection, keep the room well aired. Use air fresheners and dispose of soiled linens as soon as possible.

7. Use a sitz bath to relieve discomfort associated with a urinary tract infection.

▶ POOR URINARY CONTROL

Poor control or no control of urinary function (called incontinence) is an embarrassing condition for any person. The patient with poor control has discomfort and skin irritation from wetness, and he worries about odor and not being able to get to the toilet in time.

The incontinent person should be on a regular voiding schedule. Begin the daily routine by taking your patient to the toilet or bedside commode upon awakening in the morning. Again after breakfast, offer the toilet. Arrange the giving of fluids and toileting schedule to coincide. Your patient should use the toilet every two hours during the day and before retiring for the night.

Your schedule will be similar to the following:

7:30 A.M.	Patient arises—offer toilet
8:30	Breakfast completed—offer toilet
10:30	Morning juice break—offer toilet
11:45	Prior to lunch—offer toilet
1:00 P.M.	After lunch—offer toilet
3:00	Offer toilet
4:45	Prior to dinner—offer toilet
6:00	After dinner—offer toilet
8:00	Offer toilet
10:00	Prior to retiring—offer toilet

If your patient shows signs of gaining urinary control (or gaining continence), extend the periods between offering the toilet. However, always offer the toilet before and after meals and after your patient drinks a large quantity of fluid.

It is to your advantage to offer the toilet during the night, too. Perhaps you have noticed that your patient is dry until 2 A.M. Then by all means, offer the toilet before that time, and it may be necessary to offer the toilet again before morning. This seems like an annoying task, but eventually it may help your patient gain urinary control or even partial control. The patient will be much happier and more independent knowing he has control of his urinary function, and you will prevent skin irritation and breakdown.

Under no circumstances consider this scheduling of urine function the same as toilet training a child, and never refer to it as such. Your patient is a mature adult who warrants respect.

Some measures you can take to help your patient void are: provide privacy if possible; use a warmed bedpan or urinal; allow plenty of time; and be prompt with assistance when your patient expresses a desire to use the bedside commode or bedpan. Comfort while using the commode is important also. A daughter caring for her mother found the frail, thin woman was very uncomfortable sitting on the bedside commode. To solve this problem, she purchased a padded commode seat to replace the one on the bedside commode. The mother found this seat much more comfortable.

If you have assisted your patient to the bedside commode at a regularly scheduled time and he is unable to void, help stimulate the urge to void by turning on a water faucet. The sound of running water sometimes stimulates voiding. Still another effective measure is to place your patient's hands in a basin of warm water.

Female Incontinence

Stress incontinence is a condition that is common to females and sometimes occurs during middle age as well as the later years. The woman involuntarily expels a small amount of urine while coughing, laughing, or sneezing. Usually a sanitary napkin provides sufficient protection.

Your physician may recommend exercises to strengthen the lower pelvic muscles. These exercises are isometric and are not strenuous. They can be done while sitting, watching TV or while standing, and no one will know your patient is performing these exercises.

Before beginning these exercises, your patient must learn which muscles she will tighten and relax. Have her begin by stopping the flow of urine while voiding and then restarting the flow, noting the muscles used to stop the flow. This is one group of muscles she will want to slowly tighten and release. The other muscles to be exercised are the ones surrounding the rectal opening. The patient will slowly tighten and then release these muscles. Have her start by exercising each muscle group ten times, four times a day. Gradually, have her increase the number of exercises and continue to perform them four times a day.

The female with partial or total loss of urinary control poses a greater problem. If efforts to set up a toileting schedule are unsuccessful, you will have to use adult diapers or rubber incontinence panties. Adult diapers are disposable, and they do help keep wetness directly off the skin, but they are also expensive. Rubber or plastic incontinence panties are less expensive. They either have disposable liners, or a sanitary pad can be placed inside the panty. You also need to use linen savers and a rubber sheet covering over the bed mattress.

UNDER NO CIRCUMSTANCES USE PLASTIC GARBAGE BAGS OR OTHER PLASTIC BAGS ON THE BED. Of course, you can understand that good skin care for the incontinent patient is imperative. Change diapers and pads as they become wet, and always wash the perineal and buttocks areas with soap and water, rinsing and drying well. Zinc oxide preparations, petroleum jelly, or vitamin A and D ointment can be applied to the skin to help prevent skin breakdown. A tub bath, if tolerable to your patient, will also lessen the chance of skin breakdown. If the skin shows signs of breakdown, such as redness or irritation, despite all your efforts, consult your physician for further advice.

Male Incontinence

A male with partial or total loss of control of his urinary function will require the same meticulous skin care as the female. Special garments such as diapers and rubberized panties can be worn by males.

The Condom Catheter or External Male Catheter. Some males with poor urinary control do well wearing a device known as an external male catheter or condom catheter. This is a rubber sheathe that is placed over the penis and then connected to a drainage system. Condom catheters are available at most pharmacies and medical supply houses. Condom catheters are inexpensive and provide good protection from wetness. Furthermore, because they are not inserted into the penis or bladder, there is less chance of infection than with an indwelling (internal) catheter.

Directions for applying the external male catheter are on the package, and this procedure may vary slightly, depending on the brand used. You may have to trim some pubic hair at the base of the penis to prevent pulling. You will also need to purchase separately a drainage bag and drainage tubing to connect the bag to the catheter.

In general, the penis is washed, rinsed, and dried. A double-sided strip of adhesive, which is provided with the package, is wrapped spirally around the penis about one inch from the base of the penis. The sheathe or condom is then rolled up over the penis and secured over the adhesive strip. When applying the condom catheter, be sure the tip of the condom is about 1/2 inch from the tip of the penis, so it does not restrict the urinary flow and does provide a small receptacle for collecting urine. Some brands of sheathe catheters provide another strip of adhesive to secure over the penis, or you may use paper adhesive tape, if necessary. The adhesive strips should be secure but not tight or restricting.

To remove the sheathe catheter, gently reroll it, starting at the base of the penis and working to the tip. Then remove the adhesive strip.

Caring for the condom catheter requires some special attention for the security and comfort of the patient.

1. Inspect the penis several times daily for signs of swelling or irritation. Remove it immediately if these signs occur.
2. Change the catheter daily. Always wash and dry the penis well before applying another catheter.
3. Inspect the catheter for signs of twisting or kinking of the drainage tubing.
4. Secure the drainage tubing to the inner thigh with adhesive tape or a specially made leg strap to prevent pulling or dislodging of the catheter.
5. Replace the drainage bag at least weekly.

Urinary Dribbling. Some adult males suffer from the involuntary expulsion of small amounts of urine known as urinary dribbling. Exercises to strengthen the lower pelvic muscles, the same as used for female stress incontinence, may help. The male patient should also be examined by his physician to rule out any signs of urinary tract infection or prostate enlargement.

If the male has no objection, he can wear sanitary pads to provide protection from dribbling. Diapers and rubberized panties are also a possible solution. If the dribbling is minimal, a condom (the same as used during intercourse) can be worn over the penis, but use good skin care and inspect the penis frequently for swelling or irritation. The male would not want to wear a condom constantly, but it could be used occasionally to provide protection.

Enlargement of the Prostate. The prostate is a gland which is located just below the bladder in males. It encircles the urethra (the tube which carries urine from the bladder through the penis). The prostate gland produces a fluid which makes up part of the semen and stimulates the movement of sperm. Enlargement of the prostate is common, especially after middle age.

Due to the location of the prostate gland, it is understandable that the male patient with an enlarged prostate will have such symptoms as difficulty starting the flow of urine. He will also notice that his urine stream is thinner than usual. Later he develops a feeling of the need to void (called urgency) and has to void frequently. While voiding, the male also experiences burning at the bladder and penis areas. Urinary tract infections are commonly seen with enlargement of the prostate.

Sometimes the man, who is usually embarrassed about his condition, does not seek medical help until total obstruction of the urethra occurs and he is unable to pass urine. If his condition is severe, a prostatectomy (surgical removal of the prostate) is performed.

CHAPTER 7

ACTIVITY AND REST

▶ RANGE OF MOTION EXERCISES

Unless your physician prohibits exercise for your patient, range of motion exercises should be encouraged daily. Exercises may be prohibited for certain patients, such as the heart patient, the patient with phlebitis (blood clot), the arthritic patient, or those with fractured bones. Consult your physician before performing these exercises. Also ask a home health nurse or physical therapist to instruct you before attempting these exercises.

Range of motion exercises are exercises that put the large muscle groups and joints through their entire range of motion or range of movement daily. These exercises not only strengthen muscles and prevent muscle wasting and contractures, but they also increase circulation and keep the joints more flexible. The bed-confined patient is especially in need of range of motion exercises because of being prone to pneumonia, blood clots, and bedsores. This is particularly true of the elderly, chronically ill, and debilitated person.

Special exercises are prescribed for the stroke victim, the patient with a fracture, or the patient with other bone and muscle problems. Follow the physical therapist's advice regarding special exercises.

A good time to perform range of motion exercises is while giving your patient his daily bed bath. If the patient is able to bathe himself, encourage him to perform these exercises without assistance. Even if your patient is mobile and is fairly independent, range of motion exercises will still be helpful.

If your patient is unable to perform these exercises alone, you can assist. Perform the exercises gently and slowly, and if any exercise causes pain or discomfort, STOP. If you are in doubt about whether or not to perform range of motion exercises on your patient, consult your physician.

Start by performing each exercise three times and gradually increase this as your patient's tolerance permits, usually to ten repetitions. These exercises may be done while lying or sitting. If you must do the exercises for your patient, take care not to put any strain on joints or muscles. Support each limb by gently cupping your palm beneath the joint. For instance, support the arm beneath the elbow while performing shoulder exercises. Practice by performing these exercises on your own joints and muscles; they will be good for you, too.

Neck

Have your patient extend the head downward as if trying to touch the rib cage with his chin, and then tilt his head as far to the back as possible without causing discomfort. This exercise resembles an exaggerated nod. (See Figure 1.)

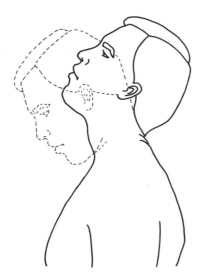

Figure 1. Neck exercise.

Shoulders

1. If possible have your patient sit erectly with back straight, rotating the shoulders forward in a circular motion, then rotating them to the back in a circular motion.

2. Shoulder shrugs are done by having your patient lift the shoulders as if shrugging.

3. Place your patient's arm at the side with the palm turned inward, and raise the arm (by supporting the elbow) to a position even with the shoulder. Then continue to raise the arm above the shoulder. You may bend the elbow during this exercise if it is more comfortable for your patient.

4. Place your patient's arm at the side with the palm turned downward, and raise the arm (again supporting the elbow with your cupped hand) slowly to a position over the patient's. (See Figures 2, 3, 4, and 5.)

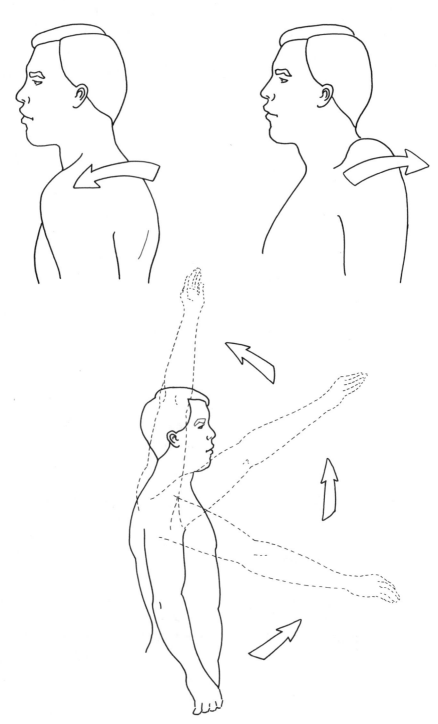

Figure 2 and 3.   Shoulder exercises.

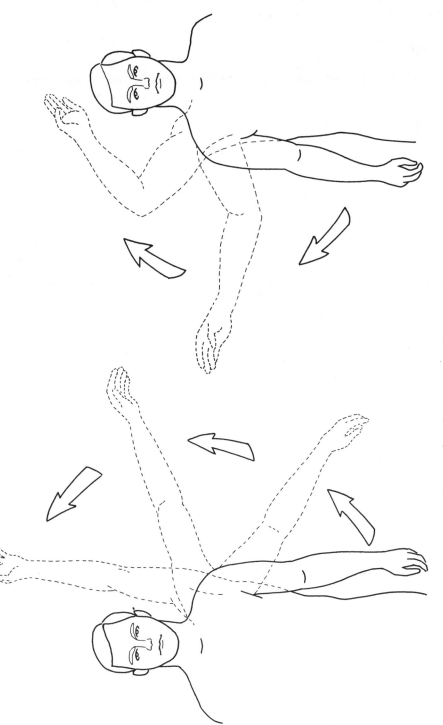

Figure 4 and 5. Shoulder exercises.

Elbow

Place your patient's arm at the side with the palm turned upward, and raise the lower arm slowly toward the shoulder. If possible, have him touch the shoulder with his fingers. (See Figure 6.)

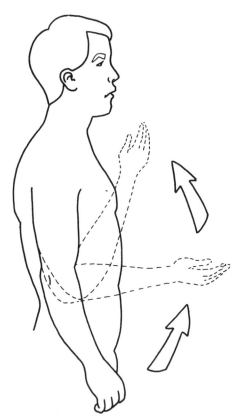

Figure 6.   Elbow exercise.

Wrist

1. Raise your patient's hand up and down in an exaggerated waving motion. (See Figure 7.)
2. You can also rotate the hand in a small circular motion, clockwise and then counterclockwise.

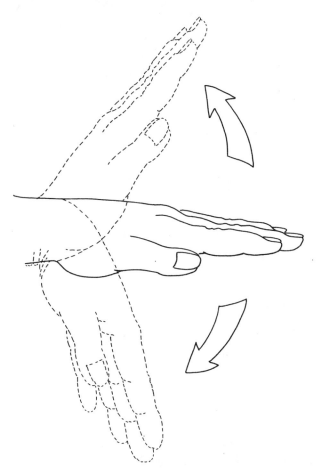

Figure 7.   Wrist exercise.

Hand and Fingers

1. Have your patient hold his fingers close together and then spread or fan the fingers.
2. Have your patient make his hand into a fist and then release it. Be sure that the thumb is exercised in this motion because the use of the thumb is very important for such tasks as eating and buttoning clothing. (See Figure 8 and Figure 9.)

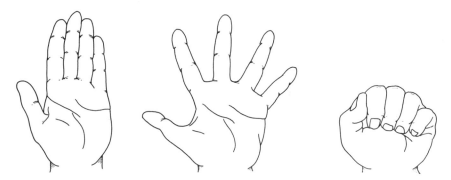

Figures 8 and 9.   Hand and finger exercises.

Hip and Knee

If your patient has had a fractured hip or hip surgery it MAY NOT be advisable to attempt these exercises.

1. Have your patient sit or lie in bed, legs aligned straight with the body, and working with first one and then the other, slide the leg along the bed away from the other leg. (Support the leg by slipping your arm underneath the calf and gently cupping the back of the knee.) Most elderly patients can only tolerate a few inches of movement to the side. (See Figure 10.)
2. Have your patient lie in bed, legs aligned straight with the body, and raise one leg from the bed and then lower it. Now flex the knee with the sole of the foot downward and then return the leg to the straight position. (See Figure 11.)

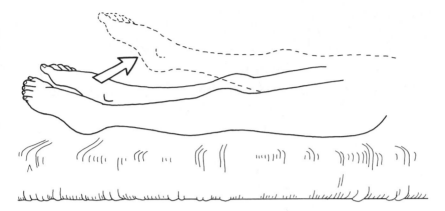

Figure 10.   Hip exercise.

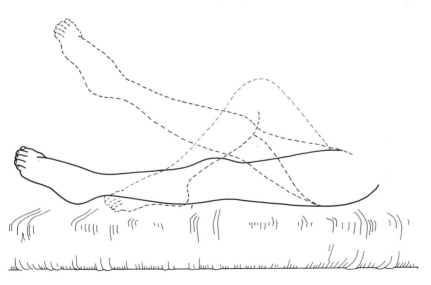

Figure 11.   Hip and knee exercise.

Ankle and Foot

1. Rotate your patient's foot in a circular motion, first clockwise and then counterclockwise.
2. Have your patient point the foot and toes upward and then downward. (See Figure 12 and Figure 13.)

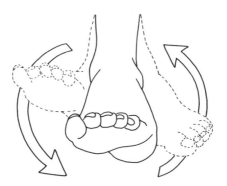

Figure 12. Foot exercise.

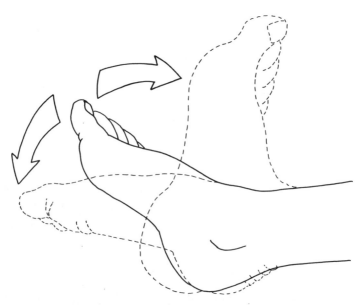

Figure 13. Ankle and foot exercise.

3. The finger exercise of spreading and fanning may also be used on the toes.

▶ GOOD BODY MECHANICS FOR THE CAREGIVER

Good body mechanics means that as the primary caregiver you will use your body to its fullest advantage for such tasks as turning, lifting, and moving your patient. Knowing how to lift your patient could very well save a personal injury and can make the task easier, safer, and more comfortable for the patient. Always ask for help if you cannot manage your patient alone. Wear comfortable, loose clothing, and low-heeled shoes when tending to your patient. Your home health nurse or physical therapist will teach you these procedures. To prevent injury or accident, use the following text as a review only after you have received proper instruction.

Turning Your Patient in Bed

If your patient's bed is adjustable, position it to a comfortable working height. Because maintaining good posture while caring for your patient is important, avoid bending over a low bed to work. You will be avoiding backache and back strain, too. Raise the side rail on the opposite side of the bed to prevent injury to your patient.

To turn your bed patient, stand on the side of the bed toward which you wish to turn the patient. Since you want gravity to help with turning as much as possible, cross your patient's far arm over the chest to the side toward which you are turning him. Now, cross the far leg over the leg near you. This distributes your patient's center of gravity to the direction in which you are turning him.

Stand close to the bed, midway between your patient's chest and hips. Standing with one foot in front of the other, place one hand on your patient's far shoulder and the other on his far hip. Get a firm grip on your patient, but be careful not to grip or squeeze so tightly that you bruise or tear delicate skin. Your nails should be trimmed to prevent injuring your patient, too.

Tell your patient that you are going to turn him and then shift your weight from the leg that is nearer the bed to your back leg as you pull the patient toward you. Use your elbows to stop your patient's turning motion, and raise the side rail before moving away from the bed. (See Figure 14 and Figure 15.)

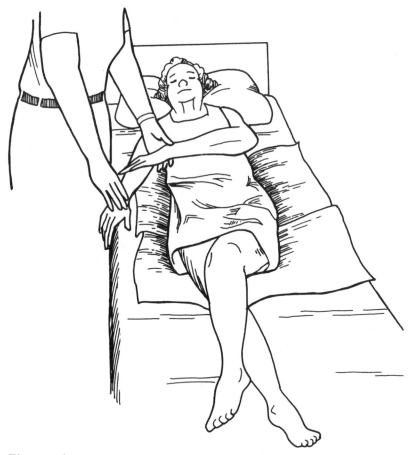

Figure 14. Using gravity to help turn the patient by crossing the arm and the leg over the body.

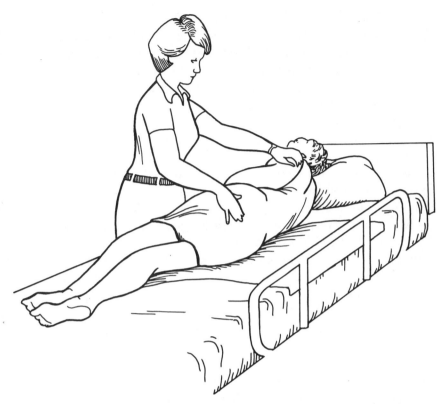

Figure 15. Turning the patient. If there is a danger that the patient will roll out of bed, you may bend at the knees and place your elbows on the edge of the mattress to stop her movement.

To turn your patient using a lift sheet, use the same principle of distributing the center of gravity by crossing his arm and leg over the body. Instead of placing your hands on your patient, grasp the far edges of the lift sheet at shoulder and hip level. Turn the patient toward you using the same body mechanics.

Moving Your Patient Up in Bed

Bed patients have a tendency to slide down toward the foot of the bed. You can prevent this somewhat by always turning the foot of the bed up slightly when elevating the head of the bed, but take care that your patient's knees are not continuously in a flexed (bent) position. A small, flat pillow can be placed beneath the knees for support. Large arteries that carry blood to the lower legs are located in the backs of the knees, and you should avoid putting undue stress on these arteries.

To move your patient up in bed, first remove the pillows and lower the head of the bed to a flat position. If your patient is able, he can assist by flexing the knees, raising the buttocks, and pushing himself with the soles of the feet which are planted firmly on the mattress.

You stand at the side of the bed with one foot ahead of the other and your body turned toward the head of the bed. If you must bend down to reach your patient, use your knees to bend, not your back. Slide one hand under your patient's shoulders and the other under the thighs. If able, your patient can assist by grasping the headboard of the bed and pulling his own weight.

In order for your patient to help as much as possible, use a signal so you will both be working together. Say, "On the count of three. Ready . . . One . . . Two . . . Three." Shift your weight from your far leg to the one nearer the top of the bed as you move your patient up. (See Figure 16.)

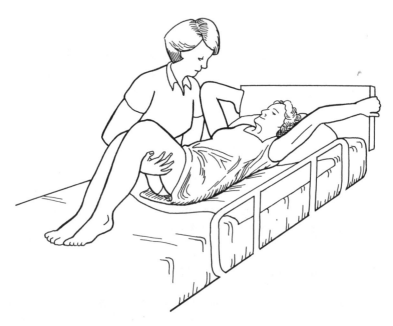

Figure 16. Helping the patient to move up in the bed.

If your patient is unable to help, you might need the assistance of another person to move him up in bed, or you can use your lift or turning sheet for this purpose. This is especially important if the patient is prone to bruising, skin tears, or bedsores.

You may also have problems with the mattress sliding down in the bed, and again you will need assistance to place the mattress in its proper position. A tightly rolled blanket or pillow placed between the mattress and the foot of the bed will prevent sliding.

Dangling Your Patient

For the patient who has been confined to bed for a long period of time, it is unwise to assume a sitting position and then a standing position without being accustomed to the change of position. Some patients become dizzy when their position is changed too quickly, and for those, assuming a sitting or standing position should be done slowly.

For the patient who has been lying in a flat position for a long period, begin getting him accustomed to sitting by raising the head of the bed for short times. Gradually increase the height and length of time the head of the bed is elevated.

If your patient tolerates the sitting position well, proceed to dangle him. Dangling might sound as if you are going to somehow suspend your patient in midair, but actually dangling means that you raise him to a sitting position on the edge of the bed with his feet out over the side. Your patient will then be sitting on the side of the bed.

With your patient lying on his side and the head of the bed raised to a 45° angle, stand facing the foot of the bed, once again with one foot ahead of the other. Slide one arm under your patient's shoulders and the other over his knees in such a way that your upper arm is over the knees and the lower portion of your arm is beneath the knees. Using a turning motion with your body and shifting your weight from front to back leg, bring your patient to a sitting position.

Place a footstool beneath your patient's feet to provide better balance if the feet do not reach the floor. Place the over-the-bed table in front of the patient so he can rest his arms on the table. You may place a pillow on the table for added comfort. If the patient becomes weak or dizzy, quickly place him in a lying position by reversing the procedure with one arm at the shoulders and the other at the legs as before.

Dangle your patient several times before you attempt to have him assume a standing position. For safety, have another person present when you attempt a standing position for the first time. Your physical therapist will help you with this. Once your patient is in an upright position, stand near—facing him. Do not attempt taking any steps until the patient is accustomed to standing. If your patient begins to fall do not try to catch him, or you will probably both fall to the floor. Instead, you can break the fall by easing the patient to the floor or to the bed if it is nearer. (See Figures 17, 18, and 19.)

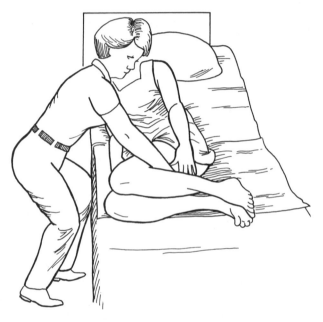

Figure 17.   Helping the patient to sit up—Step 1.

Figure 18 (top of opposite page).   Helping the patient to sit up—Step 2.

Figure 19 (bottom of opposite page).   Helping the patient to sit up—Step 3. Dangling on the side of the bed. Note that the patient's feet are placed on a footstool. An over-the-bed table could also be used for the patient to rest her arms.

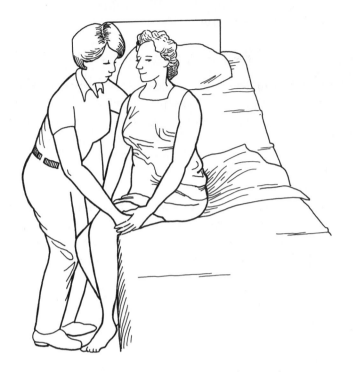

Figure 18.

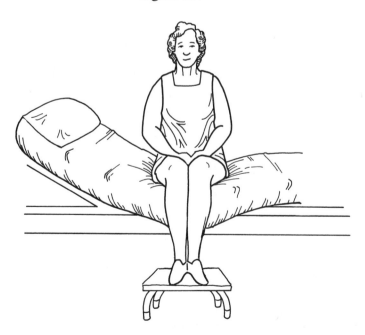

Figure 19.

Moving from a Bed to a Wheelchair

Whether transferring your patient from bed to a wheelchair, a regular chair, or a bedside commode, the same procedures apply. First, lower the height of the bed so that your patient's feet can rest on the floor. If the height of the bed is not adjustable, use a low footstool. Your patient sits on the side on the bed, dressed in shoes and robe. Place the chair directly alongside the bed with the front of the chair facing the front of the bed.

Then stand facing your patient with one foot positioned in front of the other. Have your patient place his arms around your shoulders while you place your arms around his waist. As the patient leans forward and places weight on his legs, place your nearer knee against his knees to prevent buckling. Turn and place your patient in the chair. A signal of "Ready . . . One . . . Two . . . Three" will allow him to work with you as much as he is able. (See Figures 20, 21, and 22.)

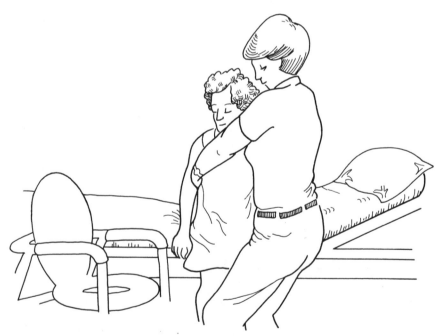

Figure 20. Transferring the patient to a bedside commode—Step 1. The bedside commode is positioned to the right of the patient, facing the head of the bed.

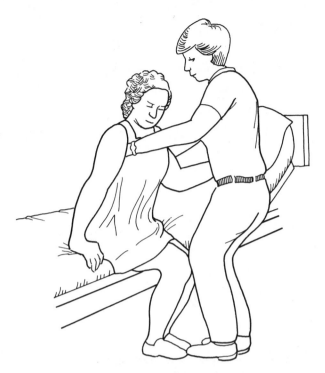

Figure 21. Step 2. Note the caregiver's knee is positioned to support the patient's knee(s).

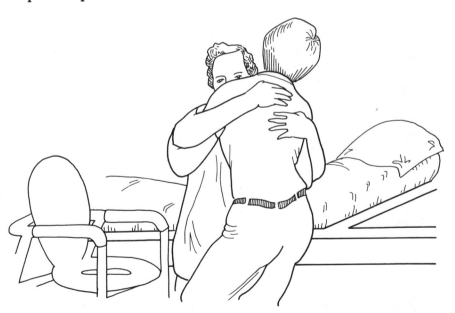

Figure 22. Step 3. Being transferred to the bedside commode.

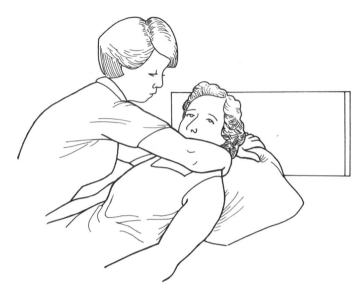

Figure 23. Fluffing the patient's pillow. The caregiver supports the patient's neck and upper shoulders with her right hand and arm, while she uses her left hand to turn and fluff the pillow.

When transferring your patient to a wheelchair, be certain the wheels are locked. Wheelchairs are available with removable armrests, which is helpful with transferring in and out of bed. The wheels of hospital beds can also be locked to prevent the bed from moving and possibly causing an accident. If there is any danger of the bedside commode sliding away from you as you transfer your patient to it, place a nonskid mat beneath the commode. Some bedside commodes are equipped with lockable wheels.

Portable hydraulic lifts are available for lifting patients in and out of bed, but be sure you have proper training in the use of this equipment before attempting to transfer your patient alone. These lifts are usually frightening to patients, and it is quite easy to have an accident if you are not properly trained in their use.

Tips for Better Body Mechanics

The caregiver may consider also some general tips for lifting and transferring your patient.

1. Bend with your knees, not your back.
2. Placing your feet in a wide stance gives you a greater center of gravity.
3. Adjust the bed to a level that is comfortable for you.
4. When lifting, hold your patient close to your own body.
5. Slide your patient whenever possible. This is easier than lifting, but be careful not to scrape his delicate skin.
6. Pulling your patient toward you is easier than pushing him away from your body.
7. If you are uncertain about lifting or transferring your patient, ask for assistance from another family member. Use common sense when attempting to lift your patient. For example, if you are five feet tall and weigh a hundred pounds, and your male patient is six feet tall and weighs two hundred pounds, you will not be able to lift him alone.
8. Encourage your patient to help as much as possible with lifting, transferring, and turning.

▶ ASSISTANCE FOR THE WALKING PATIENT

Your patient may be able to walk with some assistance. If your patient is unsteady on his feet, you can help steady him during walking by standing slightly in back with your near arm positioned around his back and your hand at the side of his waist. With your far arm you can support the elbow near you. (Sometimes it is preferred that the shoulder be supported. This will prevent the patient, such as a stroke victim, from falling forward or bending at the waist.) A special waist belt is available to help steady your patient, or you may improvise one by folding and securing a bath towel around his waist. Use heavy-duty safety pins (such as diaper pins) to secure the bath towel. Adjust the towel to fit the patient's waist snugly, leaving enough room for you to slip your hand beneath the towel to offer some support for your patient. Use a cane or walker for those with poor balance or unsteadiness. Your physical therapist will instruct you.

Your patient should wear sturdy, low-healed shoes, and should begin by walking only a few steps. Your physical therapist will give further instructions. Have a chair or wheelchair near in case the patient becomes weak or dizzy. Allow your patient to set the pace for walking, and never try to hurry him along. If possible, attach a handrail on an empty wall, such as a hallway, to allow your patient to practice walking.

Encourage your patient to stand tall while walking. The head should be held high with shoulders back, abdomen tight, pelvis tucked in, and toes should be pointed straight ahead. Your patient may have a tendency to walk with head bowed, watching each step, but you should discourage this practice. As the caregiver helping your patient move about, you should also practice good posture while walking, sitting, and standing.

Taking a Seat

Some people have a tendency to sit down by "blindly" dropping themselves into a chair. Proper instruction regarding sitting down in a chair can save unnecessary injury.

As your patient nears the chair, have him turn his back to the chair. The patient will then step backward until the backs of both legs are touching the seat of the chair. Next, the patient will place first one hand and then the other on the chair's armrests. Now the patient may safely and slowly lower himself into the chair. Chairs that are too low will be difficult to get into and out of. Motorized chairs (with seats which move up to help the patient rise from the seat and down to help lower the patient onto the seat) are available, but they are also expensive.

Encourage your patient to use good posture while seated. His back should be straight and against the back of the chair, and he should avoid crossing his legs. A footstool can be used if his feet do not rest comfortably on the floor.

The Use of Canes and Walkers

Your patient may require the assistance of a cane or a walker. If your patient uses a cane, your physical therapist will adjust the height of the cane. The shoulders should be straight with the elbows only slightly bent, about 20 degrees. (Another way to judge whether your patient's cane, or walker, is the proper height is to have him stand erect with arms at his sides. The walker or cane should be at wrist level.) A drooping shoulder means that the cane is too short, and an elevated shoulder means it is too long. A cane may be the simple straight variety used when there is only slight weakness or the quad cane—with four supports—for the weaker person or a patient with poor balance. Whatever type of cane the patient uses, be certain the rubber tips on the ends are in good condition, and replace them as necessary.

To walk with a cane, your patient will step with the cane and the weaker leg together, followed by the stronger leg. The cane should be held close to the body once the patient has mastered this technique.

Remind your patient to keep the cane at hand at all times. Do not allow him to arise from a chair by using the cane for support; instead use the armrests.

Walkers also need to be adjusted to the correct height, and the physical therapist will do this for you. To walk with a walker, your patient should advance the walker a short distance in front of him (about the length of one step) and then advance the weaker leg, followed by the stronger leg. Both feet should now be even, and the patient can advance the walker for the next step.

The person who has to use a walker continuously will appreciate a degree of independence gained by attaching a catchall carrier device across the center bar. This "pocketbook" can be made by sewing a small towel with pockets to the walker. Since it is impossible to carry objects while using the walker, your patient can now place small objects in the pockets and transport them as he walks. A purse or a small plastic shopping bag can also be used.

Folding walkers are available. They are less bulky to store and fold nicely while traveling.

▶ PROVIDING REST

The amount of resting time needed varies greatly. Heart disease, iron deficiency anemia, breathing problems, and other problems that are common to the elderly patient all increase the need for rest. For certain physical ailments, the amount of rest needed will be ordered by the physician. The ill person who is fairly independent in the home will probably still need extra rest, and you should encourage him to lie down each afternoon for at least one hour.

Some elderly patients may consider the need to rest as a sign of old age and resist their body's need, while others may insist upon too much rest because they are old. Your patient does not need to sleep during the afternoon rest period, and too much sleep during the day often spoils the night's sleep, but the rest time is important. Because most elderly tend to have swelling of their feet, an hour's rest during the afternoon with the legs elevated helps to relieve this problem.

If your patient rests a good deal of the time yet always complains of feeling tired, there may be an underlying physical problem, and this should be brought to the attention of the physician. Feeling constantly fatigued is also a symptom of depression, and this should also be brought to the attention of the physician.

Sleep

Elderly persons usually require less sleep than younger ones. The elderly person does not sleep as deeply as he once did, and his sleep is more interrupted. Consider this along with the fact that he may get up two or three times during the night to void, you can readily see why the elderly complain about lack of sleep.

Some patients like to retire early in the evening, and their sleep is then completed by three or four o'clock in the morning. If this routine does not disturb you, your family, or your patient, it is best not to change it. But if your patient complains of constantly being awake too early, help establish new sleeping patterns by encouraging him to remain awake later in the evening. Perhaps you or a family member could watch television or play a game of cards with the patient to delay bedtime. The person who has retired at exactly eight o'clock every evening for the last 40 years will not be able to stay awake until eleven. Instead, only try to delay bedtime by half an hour and gradually increase this time.

Encourage the patient who awakens very early in the morning to perform quiet activities, such as reading or listening to the radio. These activities sometimes help your patient fall asleep again.

Insomnia

Insomnia (inability to sleep properly) is a common problem of the elderly patient. Do not be concerned if your patient has an occasional poor night's sleep. However, if the problem is one that occurs frequently, take measures to aid sleep. To help improve sleeping habits, first try to discover why the patient is not sleeping. Pain, worry, or anxiety could cause sleepless nights.

After establishing a time for bed, help your patient prepare for bed by offering the bedpan or bedside commode. Encourage him to wash his hands and face, brush teeth or dentures, and use mouthwash. Be certain that the patient who wears diapers or incontinence pants is clean and dry. A back massage may be helpful. Adjust the pillows, and be certain your patient is in a comfortable position once in bed. Those with heart or lung problems will usually breath easier if the head of the bed is elevated to a comfortable position for sleep. Provide a quiet environment, and place the call bell within reach. A night-light is essential, especially if your patient will be getting up for trips to the bathroom during the night.

Steps for Promoting Sleep

Promoting a good night's sleep is helpful for you and your patient. Following are some steps for promoting sleep.

1. Provide a warm drink, such as warmed milk, but avoid stimulants, such as coffee and tea. Some patients prefer a snack before going to sleep, but this should be a light food such as a few graham crackers, gelatin, or a few cookies with warmed milk. Some patients actually awaken through the night because they are hungry.

2. The anxious or worried person will sleep poorly. Some patients tend to worry over the slightest problems. They worry about the weather even though they can stay inside during inclement conditions. They fret over their financial situation even though they may be financially secure. It is sometimes helpful just to be able to discuss these problems with someone who cares and has a loving attitude. For the constant worrier, you may have no choice but to discuss the problem with your physician, who will perhaps prescribe a mild sedative to be given before going to bed.

3. The patient with pain, whether mild or severe, will need a pain medication. For severe pain, your physician will probably order a strong pain medication, while a mild pain can probably be eased with over-the-counter analgesics such as acetaminophen. A comfortable position in bed with the pillows positioned correctly will also help.

4. Leg cramps are a common nighttime complaint of the elderly. Sometimes gentle exercise to the legs, such as the range of motion exercises, will help ease these cramps. However, if leg cramps occur often, discuss this with your physician. A low potassium level in the blood is one cause of legs cramps, and this will need your physician's attention. Other causes of leg cramps include calcium deficiencies and circulation problems. Muscle relaxants are sometimes prescribed to ease leg cramps.

5. Only as a last resort should your patient depend on sleeping medications. Usually, the elderly do not respond well to these medications. They become dependent upon medication to produce sleep, and the following day they may have a "hung over" feeling. Sometimes sleeping medications cause mental confusion and nightmares. If your patient does take sleeping medications, use them sparingly for that occasional night when the patient just cannot fall asleep, rather than on a routine basis.

▶ DIVERSIONAL ACTIVITIES

A good night's sleep often has a direct relationship with how active the person is during the day. Your patient needs as much activity as ability allows. The individual who has led an active and fulfilling working career, for example, will quickly become bored idly sitting in front of the television screen all day.

If the patient is able, encourage the performance of small chores. Even though the patient may be confined to a wheelchair, he will probably be able to dust the furniture or dry the dishes. Encourage your patient to assist with cooking, although this may mean only paring potatoes. Always praise and be appreciative of any assistance your patient can give, thus reinforcing a sense of worth and accomplishment. Everyone wants to feel needed.

If the patient is capable and weather permits, encourage daily walks outdoors. A trip to browse through a local shopping mall provides diversion as well as exercise. The patient may enjoy attending church and being active in church functions. Keeping in touch with others the patient's own age, either by visiting them or inviting them for a visit, is also important.

Letter writing is one way many persons keep in communication with friends and relatives. Mrs. S. is an example.

Mrs. S. lived far away from her friends and relatives, and she loved to write long, newsy letters to them. But eventually her eyesight failed, and her hands trembled too much to write. To solve this problem, her family purchased a tape recorder, and she recorded her "letters" on tapes and sent them to friends and relatives. Some who received her tapes used this same method of reply.

The telephone is also a source of communication your patient can employ. If your patient enjoys long talks with a friend in your immediate area, consider having a private line installed in his room. This will free your own telephone for your family's use.

Your community probably has a senior citizens activity center. Encourage your patient to take part in its functions. He may also enjoy belonging to lodges and various clubs in the community.

Less strenuous activities are needed for those who tire easily or are weak. Some of these activities could include reading, painting, collecting coins or stamps, making latch-hook rugs, and fly tying. Also consider leather crafts, small wood crafts, model ships and cars, crossword puzzles, sewing crafts, and needlework. Men should be encouraged to learn crochet, embroidery or other needlework. Many men do well at needlecrafts, and they gain a sense of accomplishment in being productive.

Mr. P., a retired coal miner, suffered from a chronic illness that left him too weak to perform any activity requiring standing or muscular activity. His wife encouraged him to learn embroidery, and although he knew his death was near, he became consumed with embroidering quilt tops. He died with a sense of accomplishment, knowing he had given each of his children and grandchildren an exquisite, heirloom quilt. In his own way, Mr. P. left behind a bit of himself and a bit of immortality—something everyone strives for.

Allow your patient to decide the sort of activities he would like to pursue. Consider hobbies or activities previously enjoyed. To insist that an elderly or any chronically ill adult male take up fishing when he would rather read a book would only lead to frustration and hostility.

Music is an enjoyable, relaxing diversion to which even the most confused person seems to respond. Tape players are easy to use and may provide hours of soothing relaxation.

Consider getting your patient a pet. The therapeutic value of pets for the older person is a subject that is just beginning to be studied. The older person gains a sense of responsibility in caring for a pet. A pet can also satisfy the need in all of us to touch and be touched in return. Avoid getting a frisky puppy or kitten for an older person, but consider a mature, trained pet. Other pets, such as tropical fish and birds, may also be enjoyed.

For the person who has always enjoyed gardening but is no longer able to tend a garden, consider houseplants, window boxes, and terrariums. Subscribe to various gardening magazines, books, and catalogs. Reading such material will not remind your patient that he can no longer perform the actual gardening; instead he will be able to keep in touch with a hobby he enjoys.

A 50-year old, Mrs. R., who had been an avid gardener, suffered from multiple sclerosis. Even though her health failed and she was incapable of strenuous physical activity, she spent long winter afternoons pouring through her collection of gardening catalogs and planning her spring flower garden. As springtime neared, she convinced her daughter to purchase a few of the plants she particularly wanted, and from her wheelchair in the backyard, she thoroughly enjoyed supervising her daughter and grandchildren in the planting and tending of her flowers. Not only was Mrs. R. proud of "her" flower garden, but her family was quite proud of their own accomplishment.

If possible, have your patient spend some time each day outside in the fresh air. This helps to promote a good night's sleep. Long-sleeved clothing and a wide-brimmed hat should be worn for protection from the sun. Sun glare may be a problem, and sunglasses should be worn. Your patient's skin might burn quite easily, but you can apply a sunscreen lotion for protection. Sitting on the porch will be enjoyable, and a screened porch will control the problem of pesky insects.

CHAPTER 8

MEDICATIONS

▶ THE PRESCRIPTION LABEL

A medicine or medication is any substance used in the treatment of disease, in healing, or the relief of pain. Although you might think of a drug as being a stronger medication, such as a narcotic or "street drug," any medication or medicine is a drug. Medications come in many forms, and the most familiar is probably the pill. When you think of a pill, you may also think of different forms of pills, such as tablets, capsules, caplets, and spansules. Medications are also manufactured in such forms as liquids, creams, ointments, suppositories, powders, foams, aerosols, and skin disks.

The physician may have ordered your patient to take several medications throughout the day, and you are a little worried about giving the correct pills, eye drops, and liquids at the correct times. Medications can be quite confusing, but with some knowledge, an understanding of prescription labels, a written schedule, and a consistent plan, you will have no problems.

There are five "rights" you should remember when preparing and giving medications.

1. The Right Person—Is your patient's name on the prescription label?
2. The Right Medication—Is this the medication that was ordered?
3. The Right Dose—Is the amount of the medication correct?
4. The Right Time—At what time(s) should the medication be given?
5. The Right Route—How are you to give the medication? This could be orally, rectally or vaginally such as a suppository, to the skin as an ointment or skin patch, or it could be drops to the eyes or ears.

The fifth right, the right route, seems simple enough. You might assume that no one could give a medication by the wrong route. However, patients have been known to insert stool softeners into their rectum because they thought a stool softener was the same as a suppository. Moreover, patients have actually chewed and swallowed suppositories because they did not know how to use them. Women have chewed and swallowed vaginal suppositories, too. Putting eye drops in the ear and ear drops in the eye is a common error; after all, the bottles look alike.

You may be wondering how these mistakes could be made. For the most part, patients and their caregivers do not take the time to read their prescription labels well. Before giving any medication, your first step is to check the label carefully. Be certain the label has the correct name of your patient and you understand the directions for giving the medication. You do not necessarily need to know the specific action of each medication, but you do need to know for what purpose the drug was prescribed. For instance, it could be for stomach spasms, for circulation, for the heart, or for infection. Your physician or pharmacist can furnish this information. If you know your patient is allergic to any type of medication (or food or other substance, such as feathers or dust), always inform your physician and always check the label for this.

The pharmacist sometimes adds special labels along with the prescription label, so be sure you understand these directions. If a medication is specifically to be taken before meals, after meals, or along with meals, this should be noted. Some antibiotics should not be taken with iron preparations or antacids because this greatly reduces the action of the antibiotic, and you need to be aware of this. Other special labels may state that you should not drive or operate machinery while taking this medication. Still others may state to drink a full glass of water with the medication. Some medications which are used to reduce fluid retention will state on the label to eat a banana or drink a glass of orange juice with the medication. (See Figure 1.)

If you are unsure about the medication or its directions, consult the pharmacist. With your physician's permission, pharmacists are now permitted to substitute generic medications in place of brand names. Some physicians approve of substituting generic medications while others do not. The advantage of a generic medication is that it is

Special Labels on a Prescription Bottle

Take medication on an empty stomach 1 hr. before or 2 to 3 hrs. after meals	Do not take dairy products, antacids or iron preparations within 1 hr. of this medication.

Pharmacy name, address, and phone number	
Prescription number	Physician's name
Patient's name	
Directions for administering the medication	
Name of medication and dosage	
Number of pills dispensed by pharmacist	Pharmacist's initials
Number of refills	Date dispensed

Number of pills dispensed by pharmacist — Pharmacist's initials — Date of original prescription

Number of refills — Date dispensed

PLEASING VALLEY PHARMACY Valley Drive, Philipsburg, Pa. 341-9908	
532686	D. Allison MD
Wanda Williams	
Take one capsule by mouth three times a day after meals until gone	
Tetracycline 250mg	
QTY 21 PJC	Orig 11/07/86
No refills	Disp 11/07/86

Figure 1. What You Find on a Prescription Label

usually less expensive than its brand name counterpart. However, the generic medication will look different than the brand name product, and this can be confusing.

For instance, if your patient has always taken a yellow fluid pill and when the prescription is refilled you discover that the pill is now a large white tablet, you will question this. Usually your pharmacist will inform you that he has given you a generic product.

You will also notice that the name of the medication has changed when a generic drug is used in place of the brand name drug, and this can be confusing, too. Patients have been known to take two different tablets of the same medication at the same time because one is labeled with the brand name and the other with the generic name. The patient has assumed that they are two different medications.

For example, suppose your physician has prescribed Bunatrol 50 mg daily, but the pharmacist has substituted the generic brand of this drug which is Diphranochamine (fictional brand and generic names). To prevent confusion, add your own information to the label. On a strip of adhesive tape, write "Generic Bunatrol 50 mg," and place this below the pharmacist's label on the bottle. Do not cover the original label, and do not place the tape on the lid of the bottle because the lid may fit another bottle and could get switched. Keep all facts you want to remember in your diary. For example, write the date and a note, "Bunatrol 50 mg was substituted with the generic Diphranochamine. Yellow and white capsule for upset stomach." In this way you will make no error administering the medication even though the capsule is different than the Bunatrol usually received from the pharmacy.

As you read the label, also look at the dosage of the medication and make certain it is the same. Some of the common dosage measurements used are milligrams (mg), grams (Gm.), teaspoons (tsp. or t.), tablespoons (tbsp. or T.), ounces (oz.), grains (gr.), cubic centimeters (cc) and milliequivalent (mEq). Do not concern yourself about exactly what a mg is. Just check your labels to make certain they are the same. If the old prescription label reads 50 mg, you will not want to give the new refill if the label reads 100 mg unless you know the physician has increased the dose. If you are in doubt about giving a medication, always consult your pharmacist.

Setting Up a Schedule for Giving Medications

Giving medications will not be a problem if only a few are ordered, but if ten or fifteen medications are prescribed daily, this can become complicated. Do not allow the large number of medications to upset you. Begin by getting from the physician a list of all the medications to be given. If your patient has recently been hospitalized, medications will be listed on the discharge summary from the hospital. Give no other medications, and if you think the physician has missed listing a medication that your patient usually takes or has taken prior to hospitalization, be certain to inquire about this medication.

With the list and all medications in front of you, make a schedule. Read all the labels carefully. You can have someone else recheck the labels with you. The home health nurse can help you make a schedule. If a medication is to be given an hour before meals and your meals are scheduled for 8 A.M., 12:30 P.M., and 5 P.M., write on a paper the name of the medication and the times 7 A.M., 11:30 A.M., and 4 P.M. A medication that is ordered "once daily" is usually taken in the morning unless otherwise directed, and you may want to give this at 9 A.M.. Medicines given "twice a day" are spaced at 12-hour intervals if possible. Thus a medication ordered "twice a day" should be given at 9 A.M. and 9 P.M., at 8 A.M. and 8 P.M., or at another hour as long as they are spaced every 12 hours.

A medication ordered "three times a day" can be given in the morning, afternoon, and evening. If the directions specifically state to give "every eight hours" (such as some antibiotics and heart medications), in order to follow these directions, you may have to awaken your patient through the night to take the medication. For example, an "every eight hour" medication may be given at 8 A.M., 4 P.M., and again at 12 midnight. You can vary the hours to start at 6 or 7 A.M., then 2 or 3 P.M. and again at 10 or 11 P.M. if this would be less interrupting to your patient's sleep.

A medication ordered "four times a day" can be given in the morning, afternoon, early evening, and again before bedtime. The hours could be 9 A.M., 1 P.M., 5 P.M., and 9 P.M. If the label states it is to be given "every six hours, four times a day," you will have to space it over a 24-hour period. This will interrupt sleep, but the purpose of spacing the medication is so that a constant amount will be present in your patient's body at all times, and this is important.

"Every sixth hour" medications can be given at 9 A.M., 3 P.M., 9 P.M., and again at 3 A.M. If your patient dislikes being awakened at 3 A.M., try to schedule the medication when he is likely to be awake through the night. If he gets up at 4 A.M. to go to the bathroom, schedule the medication throughout the day to coincide with this schedule. Your schedule for this medication would be 10 A.M., 4 P.M., 10 P.M., and 4 A.M.

When setting up your patient's medicine schedule, try to give as many medications as possible in the morning. This includes pills that are only ordered to be taken daily with no specific time indicated. You are less likely to forget giving a medication if you give it in the morning than if you wait until later in the day.

Unless your physician has told you not to give two different medications together, you can give several different pills at the same time. There is no need to take a heart pill at 9 A.M., a fluid pill at 10 A.M., and a vitamin pill an hour after that. They can all be taken at the same time. If you are in doubt about giving a large amount of medications together, ask the doctor or pharmacist.

Some medications are ordered "as needed." These include pain medications or other medications which are only given when symptoms arise. The label might state "Take one tablet every six hours as needed for pain." This means that the medication is given for pain if it occurs, but you must space the next dosage at least six hours (or the hours specified) from the previous dose. Naturally, if your patient is not having any pain, you will not give this medication.

Sleeping medication, relaxants, and other medications may specifically state they are to be given at bedtime, so these are taken before retiring for the night. Consider the following schedule summary.

Scheduling Medications Summary

Medications to be given:	Time
Once daily	at 9 A.M.
Two times a day	at 9 A.M. and 9 P.M.
Three times a day	at 9 A.M., 3 P.M., 9 P.M.
Four times a day	at 9 A.M., 1 P.M., 5 P.M., 9 P.M.
Every six hours	spaced evenly over 24-hour period (four total doses)
Every eight hours	spaced evenly over 24-hour period (three total doses)
At bedtime	prior to going to bed
As needed	as needed, spacing doses as ordered
Before meals	½ hour to 1 hour before meals (as specified)
After meals	after eating
With meals	mealtime

You can vary this schedule from the 9 A.M. schedule. For example, if administering daily medications at 8 A.M. (with four times a day medications given at 8 A.M., 12 P.M., 4 P.M., and 8 P.M.) is more convenient for you and your patient, give them at these times. For the late morning sleeper, a schedule starting at 10 A.M. (with four times a day medications given at 10 A.M., 2 P.M., 6 P.M., and 10 P.M.) is permissible.

Now that you have listed the medications and the times to be given, make a written schedule or chart for easy reference. Use cardboard to list the schedule, and you might want to describe the medication after you list it. You can also tape a sample of each pill beside its name with transparent tape. Do be careful to keep this type of schedule out of the hands of children or your patient if he is mentally confused. Figure 2 is a list of medications and the schedule laid out by the caregiver.

Besides taping a sample of each pill onto the medicine schedule, you can also note the medicine's use and the times it is given daily, such as heart pill—one time a day.

It is a good idea to prepare each morning all medications to be given throughout the day. This way there will be no question about whether a medicine has been given; if the container for a certain time slot is empty, it has been given.

Small bathroom-size paper cups can be labeled with medication times. Small dessert dishes also work well, as do empty egg cartons. Using your schedule, just place the proper pill in the proper time

Medications to be given:

1. Digoxin 0.125 mg twice a day orally
2. Dipyridamole 50 mg three times a day orally
3. Potassium Gluconate 5 mEq one daily orally
4. Hydroxyzine HCL 10 mg as needed, every six hours orally for itching
5. HCT 50 mg twice a day orally
6. Tetracycline 250 mg every six hours orally, given on an empty stomach an hour before meals or two hours after meals
7. Lorazepam 25 mg hour of sleep orally
8. Milk of magnesia three tablespoons orally at bedtime as needed
9. Multi-vitamin one capsule daily orally
10. Cimetidine 100 mg before meals twice a day orally

Figure 2A.   List of Medications.

Medication	Description	7:30 A.M.	9 A.M.	10 A.M.	4 P.M.	4:30 P.M.	9 P.M.	10 P.M.	4 A.M.
Digoxin	small yellow		✓				✓		
Dipyridamole	small white		✓		✓		✓		
Potassium	orange coated		✓						
HCT	med. white		✓				✓		
Tetracycline	yellow cap			✓	✓			✓	✓
Lorazepam	white tab						✓	✓	
Vitamin	pink oval		✓						
Cimetidine	white tab	✓				✓			
Milk of mag. if needed	liquid						✓		
Hydroxyzine every 6 hours if needed	small violet								

Mealtimes are 8 A.M., 12 noon, and 5 P.M.

Figure 2B.   Medications Schedule

compartment. If there are small children in your home, be certain to keep all medicines out of their reach and locked up if possible.

Some medications may be ordered to be taken every other day or every third day. Mark on a calendar the days these medicines are to be given. Also list in your diary when these were given.

Rules for Giving Medications Correctly

Some general rules for giving medications are important for you, your patient, and your family.

1. If you are in doubt about a medication ask your doctor or pharmacist before giving it.
2. Check to be sure the label has the right person, the right medication, the right dose, the right times, and the right route (orally, to the skin, etc.).
3. Do not remove medications from their prescription bottle or pour them from one bottle to another. If a medication is in a brown bottle, it is because it is sensitive to light.
4. Do not store medications in a heated area, such as near the kitchen range. If you notice a change in the color of a medication or if pills are sticky or melting together, do not give the medication.
5. Give medications as ordered. Do not think that because one pill works well two will work even better.
6. Pour liquid medications holding the label side up while pouring. This will prevent smearing the medication over the label. Wipe the bottle after pouring if necessary.
7. Store all medications in one place. Do not keep sleeping medications in the bedroom and others in the kitchen or bathroom.
8. Keep all medicines away from children.
9. Keep all medicines out of reach of the confused or senile patient.
10. If your patient is depressed, stay with him until you are certain the medication has been swallowed. Such a patient could decide to store a large supply to attempt suicide.
11. Never give over-the-counter preparations along with prescription medicines without your doctor's approval.

12. If your patient develops a rash, hives, wheezing, shortness of breath, or any other symptoms that leads you to suspect an allergic reaction, stop giving the medication and consult your doctor.

13. Discard all medicines you are not currently using. All medications have an expiration date, and to administer a medicine that has been in the medicine cupboard for years could do more harm than good.

14. Do not lend or borrow medications.

15. Avoid giving alcoholic beverages with medications. Consult the physician if your patient usually drinks a cocktail with his dinner, and so forth.

16. If you skip a dose of medication, do not try to catch up by giving two at the next dose.

17. Inform the doctor if your patient is taking medications prescribed by another doctor.

18. Give the complete series of medication. If an antibiotic is ordered for seven days and your patient is feeling better by the second day, you must still complete the seven day schedule, or symptoms may reappear.

▶ GIVING MEDICATIONS

Administering Oral Medications

Your patient should be sitting in an upright position to swallow medications. Most medicines can be taken with water or juice. It is easier for both you and your patient to handle pills if they are placed in a small paper cup or other small container. Offer a drink first to help wet the patient's mouth and throat. Then place the pill(s) far back on the tongue and give more fluids. Your patient should tilt his head back as he swallows.

If your patient chokes easily, ask your pharmacist if the medication is available in a liquid form. You may also be permitted to crush certain medications and add them to small amounts of jelly or applesauce. Ask the pharmacist if you can crush medications in food. If you use this method, try to follow the food with a glass of water.

In general, pills that are placed under the tongue should not be crushed. Capsules that contain time-released pellets should not be opened and crushed. If your patient is vomiting, hold all medications until vomiting has stopped. Your patient should not chew pills unless specifically ordered to do so.

The patient who is confused may pose a special problem if he refuses to take medications. Avoid being forceful if he refuses. Wait 15 or 20 minutes, and then offer the medications again. Perhaps another family member can convince the patient to take the medications. If all else fails, consult your pharmacist regarding the use of liquids or crushing pills and disguising them in food and drinks.

Sublingual Medications

The most common sublingual medications are forms of nitroglycerin which are used by the cardiac patient for angina (angina pectoris) chest pain. These tablets are to be placed under the tongue and left in place until the entire tablet dissolves. Some nitroglycerin does cause a stinging sensation in the mouth, and this is to be expected. Your patient should not drink fluids or eat food while the pill is under his tongue.

Follow the directions exactly when administering these medications. For example, the label may state to take one pill under the tongue for chest pain and repeat at five minute intervals not to exceed three doses. If your patient's chest pain has not eased after the third dose, you will need to seek medical help.

Nitroglycerin works by causing the blood vessels to dilate and by increasing the amount of blood going to the heart muscle; therefore, your patient may experience headaches since the medication may also dilate the blood vessels of the head. The headaches may disappear after a few uses, but if they are persistent or severe, consult your doctor.

Transdermal Medications

The administration of medication by placing it on the skin is a fairly new concept. The dose of transdermal medications (skin patches or disks) is absorbed slowly and steadily by the skin, and with this route of administration there is no irritation to the stomach as with oral medications. Usually, skin patches are applied to the skin one time daily. The instructions will tell you where to apply the patch, but it is commonly applied to the upper arms, shoulders, upper back, or chest. Clip the hair from the area if necessary.

Most persons apply skin patches after bathing, but some drug producers now indicate that bathing will not harm the patch. If you do apply the patch after bathing, be certain the skin is completely dry before applying it.

Do not attempt to cut a skin patch in half, and do not borrow one from a friend because the doses vary widely. If you must apply the patch for your patient, be careful not to touch the medication pad because your skin will absorb the medication. If your patient develops an irritation or skin rash where the skin patch was applied, consult your physician.

Administering Eye Drops and Ointments

All eye medication labels should specifically state FOR THE EYE or FOR OPHTHALMIC USE. Wash your hands thoroughly before inserting this medication. If your patient has an eye infection, the lashes may be matted with discharge. Remove this by gently cleansing the outer lids with a cotton ball moistened with water. Use a clean cotton ball to cleanse the other eye to avoid spreading infection from one eye to the other.

To administer eye drops, have your patient sit in a comfortable position with the head tilted backward and turned slightly to the side in which you will be instilling the drops. Your patient should look to the side away from you or look upward. Gently pull down the lower lid, and holding the medication bottle about an inch from the eye, drop the medication in the lower, inner lid. Do not drop it directly on the eyeball, and do not touch the eyelid or lashes with the medication container.

If your hand is unsteady, rest it on your patient's cheek during this procedure. Medication bottles with nose rests are available. The nose rest is placed on the bridge of the nose to steady the bottle. Ask the pharmacist about this if instilling eye drops is difficult for you.

After instilling the drops, wipe away any excess medication or tears with a tissue. Do not place any pressure on your patient's eyeball while instilling the drops. It is not necessary to rub his closed eyelids after giving the drops. (See Figure 3.)

To instill eye ointment have your patient assume the same position as for instilling eye drops. Wash your hands and cleanse your patient's

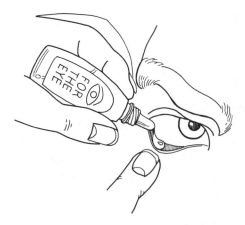

Figure 3. Instilling eye drops.

outer eye if necessary. Gently pull down the lower lid and apply a thin ribbon of the ointment to the lower, inner lid. Take care that the tip of the applicator stays clean and does not come in contact with the outer eye or any other soiled area. Have your patient sit with eyes closed for a few moments after instilling the medication. Some blurred vision may be noticeable for a short time. (See Figure 4.)

Some elderly persons complain frequently that their eyes feel dry and irritated. This may be caused by a reduction in the amount of tearing needed to keep the eyes moist, and if it is a problem for your

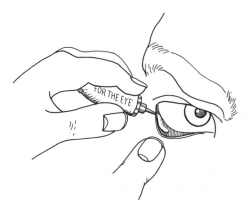

Figure 4. Instilling eye ointment.

patient, consult your physician. Special tear preparations are available for relief.

Instilling Ear Drops

Medication intended for ear use should state FOR THE EAR on the label. Warm the solution to body temperature by running warm water over the container or holding the bottle in your hands for a few minutes. Be certain the medication is only warmed to body temperature. Serious damage could result if the medication is too hot.

After washing your hands, have your patient lie on his side with the ear in which you will be instilling the drops upward. To straighten the ear canal, gently pull the outer ear slightly up and back. You may rest your hand on your patient's cheek and gently instill the specified number of drops of medication, but direct the drops to the side of the ear canal rather than straight into the ear where it could damage the eardrum. Have your patient remain in the side position for five or ten minutes.

You may insert cotton into the patient's OUTER ear canal area, but be certain to use a large wad of cotton that cannot become lost in the ear. Do not force cotton into the ear; just gently place it at the outer ear canal to prevent the medication from soiling your patient's hair or cheek.

Inserting Rectal Suppositories

Rectal suppositories are available containing medication for relief of constipation, hemorrhoids, pain, and nausea and vomiting. Suppositories containing medication for sedation are also available. The label should state TO BE INSERTED RECTALLY. Usually suppositories are stored in the refrigerator to avoid melting. If your patient is suffering from diarrhea, inserting a suppository will be of little use since it will probably be quickly expelled.

Wash your hands before starting, and wear disposable gloves for this procedure. Position your patient on his left side with knees bent. Remove the covering from the suppository and coat the tip with a water-soluble lubricant to ease insertion. Spread your patient's buttocks and identify the rectal opening. Insert the tip of the suppository into the rectum. With your forefinger placed at the end of the suppository, gently push it into the rectum, inserting it 2 1/2 to 3 inches. You will know when it is in place and when it has passed the muscles surrounding the rectum because the suppository will move on into the rectum away from the tip of your finger.

If you meet with resistance while inserting the suppository, stop and discontinue the procedure. This probably means your patient's rectum contains bowel movement, and the medication will not be effective. Of course, if you are inserting a suppository to relieve constipation, the presence of bowel movement in the lower bowel is to be expected. Encourage your patient to retain the suppository, and you may gently hold the buttocks together for a few moments if he has the urge to expel it.

Applying Ointments

Apply ointments as directed for a burn, wound, or rash. Cleanse and pat dry the area if ordered, and then apply a coating of ointment, using a cotton-tipped applicator or a tongue blade for larger areas. You may also use your fingers to apply ointments, but for the protection of both you and your patient, it is wise to wear disposable gloves, especially if the wound is infected, draining, or if there is a possibility that the rash may be contagious. Unless contraindicated, cover the area with a light dressing to keep the medication in place and to prevent the ointment from soiling your patient's clothing and bed linens. Wash your hands before and after this procedure.

Using Inhalers Properly

Medication may be given by means of an inhaler or nebulizer for the patient suffering with respiratory problems. Using an inhaler, medication in the form of a mist or vapor is introduced directly into the lungs. The container label will state how many inhalations (puffs) of the medication your patient should take and how often. The doses are metered so that each puff contains a measured dose.

To administer an inhaler properly, have your patient exhale through the nose as completely as possible, and then place the mouthpiece of the inhaler in his lips, making a good seal with the lips. Now the patient should inhale deeply through the mouth while pressing the container to release a dose of medication. After releasing the medication, your patient should hold his breath for several seconds. If you can see the medication misting around your patient's mouth, the lips were not properly sealed over the mouthpiece. If a second puff is ordered, it is best to wait at least two minutes before giving the second puff.

Respiratory medications may also be ordered by inhalation in such forms as aerosol mists or intermittent positive pressure. Ask your physician or respiratory therapist about the correct procedure for these treatments.

▶ DIURETICS

A diuretic is a medication or agent that increases the secretion of urine. The retention of fluid (swelling or edema) is the main reason diuretics are given. They are also prescribed to treat high blood pressure. Some commonly used diuretics include Chlorothiazide, Hydrochlorothiazide, Sprironolactone, and Furosemide.

The patient taking a diuretic will notice that almost immediately after taking this medication there is an increase in the amount and times of urine passed. The urine that is passed will probably be pale in color and not concentrated. Because of the need to void frequently, the patient may not want to take this medication, but it should be taken as ordered. In the case of patients suffering with congestive heart failure, the retaining of fluid could lead to heart and respiratory distress and eventual death.

Some diuretics are known as potassium depleters, which means that as they work in the body removing fluid, they also remove potassium. Your pharmacist or physician will tell you to give foods containing potassium while taking this type of diuretic. These foods include bananas, oranges, orange juice, apricots, cantaloupe, and grapes. Orange juice and bananas are the best sources. The physician will order laboratory blood tests on a routine basis to make certain your patient's potassium level is correct.

Even though some patients consume a banana or a glass of orange juice daily, they may have a low potassium level, so the physician will order a potassium supplement in the form of a tablet, liquid, or powder. The patient with a low potassium level (called hypokalemia) should take potassium supplements as ordered and continue with regular blood tests to monitor the blood potassium level. The physician will want the potassium level to be within a normal range— neither too low nor too high.

Because salt or sodium holds fluid in the body, the amount of salt allowed will be limited. If your patient is taking a diuretic, he should also follow a restricted sodium diet.

If your patient begins taking a diuretic, you may notice almost immediately that the feet and ankles are not swollen, or at least that there is a reduction in the amount of swelling. Clothing will fit better, and there will be less fluid accumulation at the abdomen. If the fluid retention was severe, breathing will be noticeably easier and there will be less shortness of breath.

In order to measure the amount of fluid your patient is retaining or losing while taking diuretics, you should weigh him daily. Weigh your patient at the same time every day, preferably in the morning, wearing the same amount of clothing. With a decrease in swelling you will also notice a decrease of a few pounds of weight. However, if your patient's weight has been stable and you suddenly notice an increased weight gain of several pounds, you will want to notify your doctor so that other measures can be taken.

▶ BLOOD THINNERS

Anticoagulants or blood thinners are ordered for the patient who has a blood clot or inflammation of a vein (thrombophlebitis or phlebitis) or the patient who is prone to developing a blood clot such as the heart patient with an artificial heart valve. Sometimes the stroke patient is also placed on anticoagulation therapy.

Whatever the reason for taking anticoagulants, it is imperative that the medication be taken as ordered. These medications alter the clotting time of the blood, and your patient will be more prone to bleeding. Coumadin® (crystalline warfarin sodium, U.S.P.)[6] is a common anticoagulant medication. When starting therapy on this type of medication, your physician will order daily blood work to regulate your patient's pro-time (prothrombin time) or clotting time of the blood. Later, if prolonged therapy is needed and the clotting times remain stable, the blood work may be ordered weekly or monthly.

Thrombophlebitis is defined as the inflammation of a vein with the formation of a clot. Some persons are more prone to developing blood clots than others. Although they may appear anywhere in the body, blood clots are more common in the legs. If you notice a redness, heat, or swelling in your patient's leg accompanied by pain in the area, suspect a blood clot. This will require immediate attention by your physician. NEVER RUB OR MASSAGE the area. Rubbing a clot may dislodge it or cause it to break up and travel to the heart, lungs, or brain where it could cause serious damage in the form of heart attack, pulmonary embolism, stroke, or even death.

Rules for the Patient Taking Anticoagulant Therapy

Extra care should be taken by a patient for whom an anticoagulant medication has been prescribed. Adhere to the following rules.

1. Take your medication as ordered and at the same time every day. If you miss a dose do not try to catch up by doubling the next dose.
2. DO NOT TAKE ANY OTHER MEDICATIONS WITHOUT THE PERMISSION OF YOUR DOCTOR. Take NO over-the-counter preparations without your doctor's permission. This includes any product which contains ASPIRIN or SALICYLATES, as these will interact with the anticoagulant and cause hemorrhage. Also consult your physician before taking laxatives or antacids.
3. Have blood work (prothrombin times) drawn as ordered.
4. Wear a medical identification bracelet or necklace which states you are taking anticoagulants or blood thinners. You can also carry a card in your wallet stating the name and dosage of medication you are taking.
5. Notify your dentist and all other physicians that you are on anticoagulant medication.
6. Maintain a consistent diet without wide fluctuations. It is especially important to avoid eating excessive amounts of green leafy vegetables because they contain significant amounts of vitamin K which has a direct relationship on blood clotting. This does not mean you have to avoid these foods, just eat the amounts you usually eat, avoiding excessive amounts.
7. Use alcohol in moderation and avoid "binge" drinking. Keep your doctor informed regarding any change in alcohol intake.

8. Take extra care while using sharp tools, avoiding them if possible. Use an electric razor for shaving.

9. Do not attempt to cut corns, calluses, or toenails with a sharp instrument such as a razor blade. Do not go barefoot.

10. Use a soft-bristled toothbrush.

11. Notify the doctor if you suffer from a fall or injury.

12. Notify your physician of any bleeding. This includes bleeding of the gums, nosebleeds, coughing up blood or blood-streaked phlegm, or bruising of the skin. It also includes blood in the bowel movement or black tarry stools and blood in the urine or a change in color (such as brown, orange, or rusty) that may indicate bleeding. If bleeding does occur, apply pressure to the site, if possible, and seek medical attention immediately.

CHAPTER 9

WHEN TO NOTIFY YOUR PHYSICIAN

▶ PAIN

Pain is the warning signal that something is wrong or about to be wrong somewhere in the body. Different people perceive pain in different ways, depending on their physical and emotional makeup and their cultural background. The muscular, macho man may be very reluctant to admit that he is in pain, but do not be surprised to find a frail, elderly lady just as reluctant to admit feeling pain. Furthermore, a slight toothache might cause only minimal discomfort to one person while another person will describe the same pain as excruciating.

Even though your patient does not admit being in pain, there are certain signals to look for. Pain will cause a tense and apprehensive appearance. Other symptoms may include restlessness, complaints of sleeping poorly, and tossing and turning in bed. The patient could also have a short attention span and an inability to concentrate.

If your patient does admit being in pain, you will want to discover all you can about the pain. What does it feel like? (Is it a dull ache or a sharp knifing pain?) Where is the pain? (Is it in the center of the chest or low in the abdomen?) Does it start in one area and move to another? (For instance, does the pain start in the chest and radiate through to the back?) How long does it last? (Does the pain come and go, or is it constant?) Did something bring on the pain? (Did eating a certain food start pain in the stomach, or did lifting a heavy object bring on chest pain?)

You will want to notify the physician if your patient is in pain; in turn, your physician will ask you or your patient to describe the pain. Pain could be described as aching, tingling, throbbing, burning, gnawing, twisting, sharp, stabbing, shooting, or crushing. Use your patient's exact words to describe the pain. For instance, the patient suffering from a migraine headache might say, "It feels like a hammer pounding in my head." The patient suffering from a heart attack might say, "It feels like a ton of bricks sitting on my chest."

Besides describing the type of pain, the physician will also want you to describe the location of the pain. Use any descriptive device you can to give the location—below the rib cage, a few inches above the naval, on the right knee, just below the left shoulder blade, or at the base of the spine, for example.

Your physician will also want to know if the pain is constant or intermittent and how long it has lasted. An aching pain may have occurred for two hours or even two days, while a sharp pain may have occurred for fifteen minutes.

A throbbing pain may exist in the lower leg while walking but cease when the patient rests. Describe any activity that may have caused the pain. For example, reaching for an object on a high shelf may have brought on right shoulder pain, or eating a bowl of spicy chili may have brought on stomach pain.

Chest Pain

Chest pain can be the result of many conditions in the body, but if your patient's pain begins suddenly and is severe, seek immediate medical help. Although every pain in the chest does not indicate a heart attack, only a physician can rule out the possibility that one is not occurring or has not occurred. It is not uncommon for a patient to complain of severe heartburn for several days before it is finally diagnosed as a myocardial infarction (heart attack). If the patient waits too long to seek medical assistance, death could result from what is only assumed as heartburn or indigestion.

At times heart pain may be referred to other areas of the body, such as the jaw, the arms (especially the left), the neck, or the back. Thus it is important to seek medical assistance for any of these symptoms. The patient suffering from an acute heart attack will probably be in severe distress. This person will have severe pain or tightness of the chest, be restless and anxious, have nausea and vomiting, perspire profusely, and be short of breath.

A pulmonary embolism (a blood clot in the lungs) will also produce sudden, severe pain in the chest. There may be a choking sensation with sudden shortness of breath and coughing. The patient will be in acute distress and will need immediate medical help.

Other causes of chest pain may include pneumonia, bronchitis, asthma, infection of the gall bladder, hiatal hernia, lung diseases such as cancer or abscess of the lung, and peptic ulcers. If your patient has recently suffered a fall, you might also suspect that chest pain is caused by fractured ribs.

Counting the Pulse. In certain diseases or if your patient is taking certain medications, your physician may ask you to check your patient's pulse daily or before giving certain heart medications. A pulse is the throbbing of an artery felt as the heart pushes blood throughout the body. Pulses are best felt where an artery is directly over a bony area, such as the radial pulse in the inner wrist. Here the radial artery passes over the radius bone. Other areas where pulses can be found include the temples, behind the knee, and the top of the foot. Sometimes you can actually see a pulse throbbing at either side of the neck at the carotid arteries.

Count the pulse rate while your patient is resting quietly, either sitting or lying down. To locate the radial pulse, rest your patient's arm comfortably in his lap, on a chair arm, or atop the bed. Using your forefinger and middle finger, find the base of the thumb, at the fatty pad, and slide your fingers slowly and gently to the inner wrist. With a little practice you will be able to locate the pulse in a few seconds.

Palpate the pulse gently without too much pressure because pressing too hard on the artery will make the pulse difficult to find and count. Do not use your thumb to palpate the pulse because your thumb has a pulse and you may feel your pulse instead of the patient's. However, if your patient has been taught to count his own pulse, he may use the thumb if desired, because he will be counting his own pulse.

To count the pulse rate, you will need a watch with a sweep second hand. Count each beat for 30 seconds and multiply by 2. This will give you the number of beats per minute. If the pulse is irregular or difficult to count, count it for a full minute. With practice you will be able to note if your patient's pulse is regular or irregular, strong or weak.

A very slow pulse rate of 60 beats per minute or below is called bradycardia. Bradycardia occurs in some diseases and is also seen if your patient is taking cardiac medication which slows the heart rate. A fast pulse rate of 100 beats per minute or over is called tachycardia. Tachycardia may occur with certain diseases.

After some experience you will become familiar with your patient's pulse, and it will be helpful to record his daily pulse in your notebook for reference. The pulse rate can vary greatly in the same patient from day to day. Do not be alarmed if your patient's pulse is usually 68 beats per minute and jumps to 84, because many emotional and physical factors affect the pulse rate. However, if your patient's pulse is usually about 70 beats per minute and then speeds to 120, tell your physician about this increase.

If the physician has instructed you to count your patient's pulse, be certain to ask what range of pulse rate to expect as normal and the low and high rate at which the doctor will want to be notified.

Abdominal Pain

Abdominal pain can be a dull ache or burning, cramping or colicky pain, or severe pain. In the case of severe pain you will need to seek medical assistance immediately. Besides stomach and intestinal disorders, abdominal pain could also be caused by bladder or kidney disorders, gall bladder and liver disorders, pleurisy, disorders of the female reproductive system (such as a cyst of the ovary or endometritis of the uterus), and disorders of the prostate in males, just to mention a few.

The patient with abdominal pain may refuse to eat, belch gas or pass gas via the rectum, have nausea or vomiting, have diarrhea or constipation, be short of breath, be feverish, or may void frequently and complain of urinary burning. Whatever the symptoms, try to give your physician the most accurate description possible.

Appendicitis is a life-threatening condition which will require immediate surgery. At times it is difficult to distinguish appendicitis from other abdominal disorders. The pain may generally radiate throughout the entire abdomen or be over the naval. For this reason it is important not to give laxatives or administer an enema to anyone complaining of abdominal pain. This could cause the appendix to burst and spill contents of the bowel into the abdomen, causing peritonitis. Use caution with any abdominal pain or other abdominal symptoms, and consult your physician for further advice.

Other Types of Pain

Arthritis is a common condition in the elderly which involves the joints. The three common types of arthritis are rheumatoid, osteoarthritis, and gout.

The patient may first only notice a stiffness of the fingers or hand when arising in the morning, but eventually there will be actual joint pain. At times the affected part may be red, inflamed, and swollen. During the acute phase when pain, joint redness, and swelling occur, it is best to rest the area and apply warm moist heat. Warm moist heat can be applied by the use of wet compresses, special heating pads which use water to conduct heat, and baths. Dry heat obtained by the use of a regular heating pad is not thought to be as effective as moist heat. USE CAUTION WITH ANY HEATING PAD ON AN ELDERLY PATIENT. Do not massage a joint that is acutely inflamed or swollen.

If your patient does desire to use a moist heating pad, keep the setting on low and inspect the area routinely for any signs of redness or burning. To treat back pain, have the patient lie on his stomach or side with the heating pad applied over the back. Do not allow your patient to lie on a heating pad or position it beneath him.

Both rest and exercise are prescribed for the arthritic patient, and the physician will advise you on a program for your patient. Many drugs are used for the treatment of arthritis and should be taken as ordered. Some of these medications may cause upset stomach. If your patient's prescription label states that it is to be taken with food, give it with meals or in the evening with a nighttime snack. If your patient complains of upset stomach even though you have taken these measures, notify your physician.

▶ RESPIRATORY DISTRESS

Many diseases, including congestive heart failure which is common in the elderly, can cause respiratory distress or shortness of breath. Usually your patient will be able to tell you that he is having difficulty breathing. Some elderly patients develop shortness of breath with exertion such as walking up the stairs. Observe your patient's skin color. Cyanosis (bluish tinge to the skin) is sometimes noted with shortness of breath, or the skin may have a dusky or grayish cast. The nailbeds, lips, and ear lobes, are good indicators to alert you of cyanosis.

Some persons may have difficulty breathing while lying in bed. Such a patient needs several pillows under the head or the bed adjusted to a sitting position. Doctors commonly ask patients how many pillows they need to use on their bed in order to breathe easier. If your patient has not needed extra pillows but suddenly develops this need, notify your physician.

The patient with acute respiratory distress will be very frightened. He may be gasping for air and feeling as though he is going to suffocate. If this occurs, try to reassure your patient and help him to a sitting position to aid breathing. If possible, have another family member summon an ambulance or other medical personnel, such as paramedics, while you remain with your patient. Both you and your patient will be frightened, but try to remain calm until help arrives. Some patients suffering with respiratory diseases do keep an emergency supply of oxygen in the home, and you will give your patient oxygen if it is available. Learn how to use this equipment before an emergency arises (see Chapter 12).

Coughing is another sign that your patient is having or developing a respiratory problem. A cough may be described as dry and hacking. A cough is called productive if mucus or phlegm is brought up from the lungs. The sputum (or mucus or phlegm) that is produced should be observed for amount, thickness, and color. Normal sputum is clear in color. If you notice that your patient's sputum has changed to thick milk white, is yellow, green, pink, blood tinged, or foamy, you will want to notify your physician.

Pneumonia is common to the patient who is confined to bed, but there are measures you can take to help prevent this complication. Encourage your patient to get out of bed or dangle at the side of the bed if permitted by your physician and if his condition will tolerate this. Change body position at least every two hours, and encourage the patient to take deep breaths and cough to clear the lungs. Offering fluids, especially water, helps your patient to bring up phlegm. Milk and milk products sometimes cause an increase in the amount of phlegm produced. If your patient is having difficulty with phlegm, you may want to eliminate milk products until the condition improves.

Patients who have recently had chest or abdominal surgery and those suffering from fractured, cracked, or bruised ribs are also prone to developing pneumonia. They tend to take short, shallow breaths because deep breathing causes pain in the incision or injured area; however, encourage your patient to take deep breaths. Support the incisional or injured area by bracing it with a pillow or folded towel while the patient takes deep breaths and coughs.

Counting and Observing Respirations

Evaluating your patient's breathing pattern can easily be done while checking his pulse. Count the number of times the chest rises with inspiration in 30 seconds and multiply this by 2. This will give the total number of respirations per minute. If the respirations are difficult to count, count them for a full minute. You may also place your hand over your patient's chest and count the number of inspirations (or rises of the chest) if it is difficult to see them.

While counting your patient's respirations, also note the depth of the respirations. Are they shallow, of a normal depth, or deep? An adult's usual respiratory rate is 12 to 18 per minute.

▶ BLEEDING AND DISCHARGES

Your physician will want to know if your patient is bleeding or losing other types of fluid from the body. Other types of fluid include the oozing of drainage from a wound, vaginal discharge, vomiting, or diarrhea.

The bleeding patient will need immediate medical care, but once you have reached the emergency room or clinic, the physician will want some idea of how much blood was passed prior to your arrival. To describe the amount, state it in measurements, such as $1/2$ cup or $3/4$ cup, or say it soaked through three washcloths, or it soaked two sanitary napkins, in the case of vaginal bleeding. If the amount is slight, describe it as a few spots or droplets, or say it was the size of a dime, a quarter, or a half-dollar.

Try to be accurate when describing the color of blood. Blood oozing from a wound may be mixed with watery discharge. It could be described as pink, watery, blood tinged, or brownish. If a dressing is in place over a wound, you can describe the size of the dressing. For example, say that a four-by-four inch dressing was soaked through with pink tinged, watery fluid.

You can assess the amount of vomitus (vomiting) if your patient vomited in a basin. Describe it as accurately as you can, such as 1/4 cup. The physician will also want to know what type of vomitus was present. Although it may be an unpleasant task to examine vomitus, knowing the type of vomitus can give your physician a clue to its cause. Vomitus can be described as clear, watery, undigested food; yellow or greenish as with bile; or bloody. Blood in vomitus can be frank bright red, or it can resemble coffee grounds.

Most persons are nauseated prior to vomiting, but if your patient is unaware that he is going to vomit and suddenly expels vomitus with a propelling force, bring this to your physician's attention. This is called projectile vomiting and is sometimes a symptom of a head injury or other disorders. Describe the type (color and consistency) and amount of vomitus. If the odor is peculiar, describe that, too.

It is sometimes necessary to describe bowel movement. This may also be an unpleasant task, but again it provides the physician with needed information. You can describe a stool as being well formed, a semisoft or mushy stool, hard and dry, pasty, or liquid. Stools are normally brown in color, but they may also be clay colored in certain conditions. Greenish and frothy stools are present in certain bowel diseases, and black and tarry ones are seen with the presence of bleeding or with the use of iron preparations. Bright blood may be present with the stool. Also note if there is any mucus or pus present. Describe the amount, color, consistency, and number of bowel movements.

Since a great deal of fluid can be lost through the body by perspiration, your doctor will also need to have some idea how much your patient perspired. If your patient was perspiring in such a manner that "sweat was pouring off," you can describe it as profuse perspiring. It will be helpful if you can also state such factors as how many times the patient's clothing or bed clothes had to be changed or that his pillow was soaked with perspiration. The skin may feel cold and clammy or warm and clammy when your patient is perspiring.

If your patient has a wound, sore, or a draining incision, it is important to evaluate and describe the type, color, and amount of drainage present. A wound discharge could be described as thin and watery or thick and containing pus. Colors vary. The amount can be described the same way as the amount of blood is described. State the number and size of dressings soaked or the size of drainage such as a quarter-size spot.

▶ CHANGES IN MENTAL BEHAVIOR

You will want to inform the physician of any change in your patient's mental behavior or personality. The person who is usually happy but suddenly becomes sad and melancholy needs a complete medical evaluation. However, some signs of mental changes are not as obvious as others. The person who stares off into space even though you have called his name three times could be labeled as hard of hearing, when really he was having a petit mal seizure (a small seizure or convulsion).

Your doctor will want to know any change in mental behavior. These changes include sudden confusion, failure to recognize old friends or family, sleeping a great deal of the time, or sleeping very little. Report any personality change which deviates from the normal.

▶ INFECTION

Infection is the invasion of the body by organisms capable of causing disease. A chronic infection progresses slowly and may last a long time, while an acute infection begins rapidly and is of a short duration. Some of the more common causes of infection are bacteria, viruses, fungi, and parasites.

Signs and Symptoms of Infection

Certain signs and symptoms are warnings of infection. If you suspect your patient has an infection, look for the following symptoms:

1. Pain—as would occur in an earache with a middle ear infection
2. Heat—such as fever or the warmth felt at the location of a boil
3. A redness or swelling—such as in phlebitis
4. A disorder in the function of a part—as painful voiding when a urinary tract infection is present.

The normal body temperature ranges from 97°F to 99°F, although the normal oral temperature is usually stated as 98.6°F. The patient with a fever may have a flushed face and hot, dry skin, a poor appetite, chills, nausea and/or vomiting, and diarrhea or constipation.

The patient may also ache all over and pass highly colored (concentrated) urine.

Any fever should be reported to your physician. The patient with a fever will require plenty of rest. To promote comfort, change bed linens and clothing as needed. Your physician will probably recommend that fluid intake be increased and drugs such as aspirin or acetaminophen be given to help reduce the fever. If your patient is suffering with chills, provide extra blankets. Warm the blankets first by placing them in a clothes dryer for a few minutes.

Taking Your Patient's Temperature

Taking Your Patient's Oral Temperature. Temperature can usually be taken orally; however, if your patient is confused or disoriented, it is best to use the rectal or axillary (under the arm) route. If the patient is resistive to having his temperature taken, wait until another time; injury could result with the use of a glass thermometer.

The oral reading will not be accurate if your patient breathes through the mouth constantly (known as a mouth breather) or is using nasal or mask oxygen. If your patient has recently eaten food, drunk liquids, chewed gum, or smoked a cigarette, it is best to wait for 20 to 30 minutes before temperature taking.

Be certain the thermometer is shaken down before inserting (96°F or below). Place the clean thermometer under your patient's tongue. Instruct him to close his lips around the thermometer, but not to bite down. Leave the thermometer in place for at least three to four minutes. Read the instructions provided specifically with your thermometer since the time may vary. Remove the thermometer; you may wish to wipe it with a tissue before reading it.

To read the oral thermometer, hold the end opposite the bulb tip introduced into the mouth with your thumb and forefinger and raise it to eye level. You should be in a well-lighted room, but it is not necessary to place it near a lamp. Slowly rotate the thermometer until a clear line appears. With practice you will be able to do this in a few seconds. Record the reading and the time in your notebook.

To shake down the thermometer, stand well away from objects in the room, and holding the thermometer opposite the tip inserted into the mouth, make a downward motion with the arm, ending with a flick of the wrist. Several of these downward motions may be needed to lower the mercury.

Thermometers can be washed with soap and cool water and then rinsed well in cool water. Soak the thermometer in a disinfectant solution, rinse and dry well, and return it to its case for storage. Store it in an area away from heat and direct sunlight.

Taking Your Patient's Rectal Temperature. Those who are unconscious or confused, are mouth breathers, or are on oxygen therapy will need to have their temperature taken by a route other than oral. You may choose rectally or axillary.

The tip of the rectal thermometer is stubby compared to the oral thermometer and less likely to cause injury to the rectum. With your patient in bed in a side position, expose the rectal area and cover the upper and lower body to prevent embarrassment and chills. Apply about a quarter-size amount of lubricant onto a tissue or a paper towel. A water soluble sterile lubricant is available, or you may use petroleum jelly. Roll the bulb tip of the thermometer in the lubricant to cover about two inches of the thermometer. Identify your patient's rectal opening by raising the upper buttocks, and gently insert the thermometer about 1 1/2 inches into the rectum. If you meet with resistance or your patient complains of pain, stop and discontinue this procedure.

To prevent injury or "losing the thermometer," which could cause serious damage, remain with your patient and hold the thermometer in place while taking the rectal temperature. Gently remove the thermometer after three minutes. Use a tissue to wipe the tip of the thermometer and also cleanse your patient's rectal area of any bowel movement or lubricant. Read, shake down, and cleanse the thermometer as with an oral thermometer.

Of course, under no circumstances would you want to use a rectal thermometer for an oral temperature once it has been used for rectal temperature taking. Also, be sure you use a stubby (blunt) bulb tip thermometer for rectal use. Clear plastic disposable thermometer covers are available to place over the thermometer, which makes cleaning up easier.

Taking Your Patient's Axillary Temperature. You may also choose the axillary route for temperature taking. If your patient is perspiring, dry the underarm before proceeding. Place the thermometer along the armpit, holding it in position until you cross the lower arm over the chest and place the upper arm close to the side of the chest. Leave the thermometer in place five to six minutes. The axillary temperature takes longer because you are not really introducing the thermometer into a body cavity. Remove, read, and cleanse the thermometer as with an oral thermometer. (See Figure 1.)

Digital thermometers are now available, and if you have problems reading a mercury thermometer, this type of thermometer will be invaluable to you. Follow the directions carefully. Disposable covers are usually available for these thermometers. Generally, the reading time is also less, and some record in thirty seconds.

Reading the Thermometer. Most mercury thermometers have an arrow marking the normal temperature of 98.6°F. The Fahrenheit mercury thermometer measures from 94°F to 106°F. (See Figure 2.)

The longer lines represent a degree such as 95, 96, and so forth. Between each longer line (whole degree) are four smaller lines to give a more accurate measurement in tenths of degrees. Count each smaller line as .2 degrees or $^2/_{10}$. These are .2, .4, .6, and .8. If the mercury registers between the lines, round it off to the next highest tenth.

Centigrade thermometers are also available. The normal centigrade temperature is 37°C. To convert centigrade readings to Fahrenheit, multiply the centigrade reading by $^9/_5$ and add 32 ($F = ^9/_5 C + 32$).

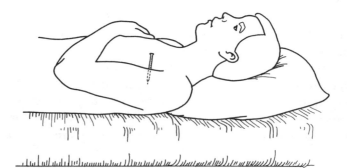

Figure 1. Taking an axillary temperature. Note the position of the arm crossed over the chest.

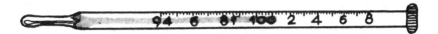

Figure 2. Reading a thermometer. This Fahrenheit thermometer reads 101.2 degrees, stated as one hundred and one point two. Some thermometers are color coded. A blue end indicates it is for oral use, while a red end indicates rectal use.

Rectal temperatures are one whole degree higher Fahrenheit than oral temperatures. Thus a rectal temperature of 101.2°F would be 100.2°F orally. On the other hand, axillary temperatures are one degree lower than an oral reading. Thus an axillary temperature of 101.2°F would be 102.2°F if taken orally.

When reporting patient's temperature to your physician, state whether you have taken the temperature by mouth, rectally, or axillary. Remember: The normal oral temperature is 97°to 99°F; the normal rectal temperature is 98°to 100°F; the normal axillary temperature is 96°to 98°F.

Measures to Control the Spread of Infection

Controlling infection and the spread of bacteria is actually a matter of practicing common sense and cleanliness of yourself, your patient, your family, and your home. Here are some suggestions to prevent the spread of infection.

1. Clean your patient's room routinely with a disinfectant solution.
2. Change complete bed linens at least once a week, cleaning bed frame and mattress with a disinfectant solution.
3. When removing linen from the bed, fold all soiled linen into the center of the bed, and refrain from shaking dirty sheets and blankets.

4. If your patient or a family member has an infection, wash all bed linens and clothing separately with a disinfectant solution added to the laundry detergent. Wash dishes in very hot water or the sani-wash cycle of your dishwasher, or use paper plates.

5. If you, the caregiver, have an open sore or cut, cover it with a plastic adhesive strip or a dressing while caring for your patient.

6. Wash all utensils in soapy water weekly and then soak in a disinfectant solution. This includes bedpans, urinals, and basins.

7. Open windows and air out the sickroom routinely if possible. Air conditioning also helps to circulate air. Clean the air conditioner filter as needed.

8. Tape a paper bag to the side of the bed for your patient to dispose of all soiled tissues. Empty wastebaskets daily.

9. Encourage your patient to cover the nose and mouth when coughing or sneezing.

10. Discourage visitors from seeing your patient if they have an infection, for example, a cold, virus, or influenza.

11. Place soiled disposable diapers in plastic garbage bags, seal, and place in a covered garbage can, preferably out of doors, until collected.

12. Use disposable items when available, such as paper towels instead of hand towels for hand drying.

13. Empty bedpans and urinals immediately after use.

14. Wear an apron to protect clothing while caring for your patient.

15. Do not hesitate to wear disposable gloves while caring for your patient, especially while cleansing the perineal or rectal area.

16. You and your patient should keep short fingernails. Clean them with an orange stick as needed.

17. Last but most important: BE A HAND WASHER. This includes you, your patient, and other family members.

▶ FLUID RETENTION

Fluid retention, also known as edema or swelling, is the accumulation of fluid in the body tissues. Edema of the feet and ankles is a common condition of the elderly, and usually this is where fluid accumulates if your elderly patient is up and walking about. But if your patient is confined to bed, you may notice an accumulation of fluid in the sacral area (lower back). The skin will be puffy and soft to the touch. At times it takes on a shiny appearance.

Fluid that accumulates in the lungs will be more difficult to notice. Your patient may have a dry cough, especially at night, and be short of breath. In severe cases respirations will sound moist or noisy.

Fluid may also gather in the abdomen, and your patient may complain of a full feeling around the abdomen, which will make breathing difficult. You may only notice that the patient's clothing is becoming tighter and you have to adjust belts and waistbands.

Fluid retention or edema is classified as pitting or nonpitting. To evaluate your patient's edema, press the ball of your finger into the swollen area and hold it there for five seconds. Release your finger and notice whether it has left an indentation or pit in the area. Pitting edema can be described as slight, + 1, + 2, + 3, or + 4 for the deepest and most severe pitting.

Nonpitting edema will feel very firm to the touch, and pressure with your finger will leave no indentation or pit because the area is so filled with fluid it can not move when pressure is placed on it.

Notify the physician if you notice any type of edema (swelling). You will also want to weigh your patient, for there will probably be a weight gain. Your physician will perhaps restrict the amount of salt in your patient's diet and prescribe a medication to reduce the edema.

Your patient also will need to rest frequently. If his feet are swollen, the patient should rest with the feet elevated several times a day, but be sure he changes position frequently to prevent pressure sores. Elevate the legs by placing them level with the hips. This is done by assuming a sitting position in bed or on the sofa or by sitting in a recliner. A low stool a few inches off the floor is not enough elevation. (See Figure 3.)

Congestive Heart Failure

Congestive heart failure occurs as a result of many different forms of heart disease, and it usually develops gradually. Common in the older adult, this condition is usually caused by an accumulation of factors. With arteriosclerosis (hardening of the arteries) and atherosclerosis (fatty deposits) in the walls of the arteries, the heart must pump blood

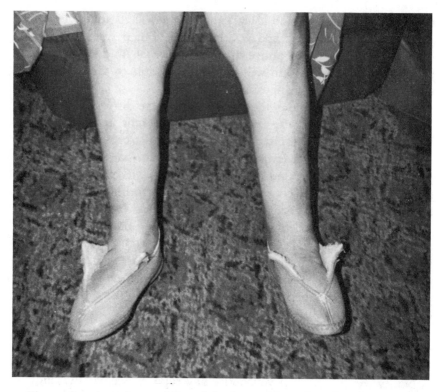

Figure 3.   A patient with pedal edema. Note that the slippers have been cut to allow for the swelling of the feet.

through narrow and inelastic blood vessels. The heart itself is also showing signs of aging, such as narrowing of the valves, and in time it cannot withstand the body demands.

A person suffering with congestive heart failure may complain of tiredness and may become short of breath with increased activity. There may be difficulty breathing while lying flat, and it might be necessary to use two or three pillows to sleep. Swelling of the feet and ankles, especially pitting edema, is a common symptom. As the condition worsens, swelling of the thighs and abdomen is also noticed. Fluid also begins to collect in the lungs, and the patient becomes more short of breath with a persistent cough. Left untreated, this condition will eventually cause death.

Treatment consists of rest, a low salt diet, and diuretics to help remove excess fluid. Heart medication is usually ordered to give the heart slower, yet stronger beats. Oxygen is given if there is respiratory distress.

Thus you can understand why observing your elderly patient for signs of weight gain and swelling is so important. In most cases if treatment is started at the first signs of congestive heart failure, the patient is spared an acute illness and respiratory distress.

If your patient suffers from high blood pressure (hypertension), it will be to your advantage to be able to monitor his blood pressure daily. You can purchase blood pressure machines at any local pharmacy. Most kits have step-by-step instructions for taking the blood pressure, and it is an easy procedure.

As mentioned throughout this book, your daily diary will also prove invaluable. Besides noting your patient's temperature, pulse, respirations, weight, and so forth, you can also note changes in medications, doctor's instructions, medications given on an as-needed basis, bowel movements, appetite, fluid intake and output, skin rashes, or anything you may want to refer to in days or weeks to come. (See Figure 4.)

Knowing how to count your patient's pulse and respirations; take his temperature; and describe pain, swelling, coughing, and types and amounts of discharge and bleeding will give you much confidence in communicating with your physician and in caring for your patient. Your confidence will bring your patient better health and comfort.

DAILY DIARY

Saturday, Dec. 6

TPR 98^2-80-16   Wt. 144 lbs. at 7^{30} AM
Ate small breakfast - nauseated
2 T. antacid given at 8^{10} AM
Voided X 2 BSC
7^{15} PM Mild mid-chest pain. Nitroglycerin tab-
    given - pain gone few minutes
All regular meds. given.
Slight swelling of feet in evening
No BM today
Incontinent of urine X 3

Sunday, Dec. 7

TPR 976-76-18   Wt. 143 lbs at 7^{30} AM
Picked at lunch.
Drank glass of Ensure at 3 PM
Headache at 4^{10} PM 2 Acetaminophen given - helped
Voided X 6 BSC
No BM today. Nauseated at X's
3 Tbsp. Milk of Magnesia at bedtime
Refused night snack
Dr. appointment Tuesday - ask about nausea

TPR- Temperature, pulse, and respirations
BM- Bowel movement; X- times; BSC- Bedside commode

Figure 4.   Example of a Daily Diary.

CHAPTER **10**

BEHAVIOR AND EMOTIONAL PROBLEMS

...

▶ FACTORS INFLUENCING THE ELDERLY

In addition to physical problems, the elderly relative now living with you and your family may experience some behavior and emotional problems. Dealing with the emotional problems of your elderly family member may be more difficult than dealing with physical problems. However, understanding some of the physical and emotional factors your patient has to deal with every day might explain why he is sometimes quiet or withdrawn and refuses to take part in a family activity.

The Physical Factors

1. The elderly are more prone to falls and accidents. This is caused by poor vision, a slowed reaction time, and not being able to adjust to a change in situations as easily as they once did. They have poor balance and less agility.
2. The older person generally tends to lose weight and may suffer from poor nutrition. Poor condition of the teeth or dentures,

gum disease, a decrease in the sense of taste, a slowed digestion process, and constipation all contribute to poor eating habits.

3. Skin becomes wrinkled and is drier. The body does not adjust to changes in heat and cold as it once did. The hair becomes thinner, drier, and gray. Nails often become thick and brittle.

4. Muscular activity is lessened; the abdomen sags, and the spine may become rounded. Strength generally lessens.

5. The total amount of bone mass decreases with age. This may cause a bent posture and an actual loss in total height.

6. Lung capacity is decreased.

7. Heart and blood vessels show signs of hardening and thickening. High blood pressure and heart disease may become a problem.

8. Sleep patterns change, and the older person tends to be a lighter sleeper. He may need more rest than he once did.

9. Sense of hearing may be decreased.

10. Kidneys undergo changes attributed to old age. There may be poor control of urinary and bowel functions.

11. Sex organs undergo changes. For the female the labia may flatten, and vaginal lubrication is diminished. The male genitals sag more, and the testicles are smaller and less firm.

12. The older person may have difficulty adjusting to new surroundings, become mentally confused easily, and experience memory loss—especially of recent events.

With these factors in mind, consider the older person suffering from physical illness. He may be confined to a wheelchair or have to use a cane. He may have to follow a medicine schedule or be on a special diet. He may become short of breath after walking 20 feet or suffer from the pain of arthritis. It is easy to understand why old age is sometimes referred to as "the season of losses."

The Emotional Factors

1. The older person must adjust to retirement, and consequently, he may feel that he is no longer a worthwhile person. With retirement, finances and living on a fixed income become a problem. The older person now has more free time than he has

ever had, but too much free time can lead to feelings of useless-
ness and poor self-esteem.

2. The older person may now have to be dependent upon others
   and may feel he is a burden.

3. Loneliness becomes a problem. The older person has usually
   seen many friends become ill and die and may have also suffered through the death of a spouse.

4. Although he may feel comfortable with old friends, the elderly
   person has difficulty adjusting to new friends.

5. The older person may no longer be permitted to drive. Traveling is more difficult, and he is unable to visit old friends and
   socialize.

6. Inevitably, the older person must face feelings about his own
   death.

With all these physical and emotional factors in mind, give deep
thought to the older person now residing in your home. Probably most
of the physical and emotional factors listed have influenced your
patient in one way or another.

Perhaps your patient is also suffering from a chronic illness, such as
congestive heart failure or emphysema. Chronic illnesses are long and
drawn out; sometimes the illness is partially under control, but at
other times symptoms of the illness flare up. Both you and your
patient will have difficulty understanding the course of a chronic
illness. There may be good days and bad days for both of you. At
times the chronic illness will take such a toll on your patient's health
that you will slowly watch his condition deteriorate before your eyes.

▶ DEALING WITH DEPRESSION

Depression is a common problem of the elderly. It is understandable
that an elderly person, especially one suffering with a chronic illness,
might be prone to depression. Consider the case of Mrs. L.

Seventy-five-year old Mrs. L. resides with her son and his family. She
suffered a stroke five years ago and is only able to walk with the use of
a walker. She has severe hardening of the arteries of the heart and

frequently has episodes of angina pain. Recently Mrs. L. became very irritable, and at times she refused to eat, saying, "I just don't feel like it." She complained to her son that he was neglecting her although he spent as much time as possible with her. She cried easily, was withdrawn, and seldom smiled. She lost ten pounds in one month.

Although it was an effort, Mrs. L. had always prided herself before in her physical appearance and was particular about her hairstyle and choice of clothing. With this recent change, however, she refused to dress, wearing her bathrobe all day long. Some days she did not bother to comb her hair.

Mrs. L.'s son was worried about his mother's emotional state. Although he did not realize it, she was showing many of the symptoms of depression. He asked his physician for assistance, and a mild antidepressant drug was ordered for his mother. The physician also explained some other measures Mrs. L.'s son could employ to help reverse this depressed state.

Mrs. L.'s son set up simple tasks which his mother could perform, such as meal planning and helping peel and chop vegetables for meals. His mother had always enjoyed washing the dishes, but with all her illnesses and the paralysis of her arm since her stroke, he assumed she could no longer handle this task. Now, after lunch each day he places two dishpans (one for washing and one for rinsing) on the kitchen table, and Mrs. L. is very pleased with herself because she can sit at the table and wash and dry the dishes. This task sometimes takes two hours, but she does not mind.

Mrs. L. was also encouraged to dress daily, and eventually her physical appearance improved. Now she is permitted to make her own decisions about what clothing to wear. She helps with family decisions, and her son often asks her opinion about family problems. Prior to this, Mrs. L.'s son thought his mother had enough problems of her own without burdening her with others, but his mother now feels more included in the family since she is consulted about minor problems. Mrs. L.'s condition has improved, and she now feels that she is a worthwhile person with a purpose in life.

Not all problems of depression can be as easily solved as Mrs. L.'s. However, it will help to set up a routine schedule which includes some activities and daily tasks. Consult your physician and be certain that all physical problems are cared for as much as possible.

Mental health counseling may be needed. Investigate whether these services can be furnished in the home in your community. Most persons, especially the elderly, are wary of seeking mental help. To them, this might be a sign that they are "crazy." Your family's attitude about mental health and illness will greatly influence your patient's decision to seek needed help. Always treat your patient with respect.

The elderly do commit suicide. Some hints that your patient is considering suicide may include statements such as, "I'm a burden to my family," "I'm tired of living," or "I'd be better off dead." Some patients might tell caregivers they are thinking of taking their life, but others will not. Do not be afraid to ask your patient if he is thinking of suicide. You can ask, "Are you considering suicide?" or "Have you ever thought of taking your own life?" This will not give your patient the idea that he should consider suicide; instead it will give him the opportunity to discuss his problems. His reply might be, "Oh, no. I'd never take my own life," or "Yes, I have thought about it, and maybe it's the only answer."

If your patient's reply is the latter, take immediate, appropriate measures. Notify your physician and have arrangements made for a mental health evaluation. In most areas a mental health crisis telephone number is available for emergency situations. Never take a person's threat to commit suicide lightly. In some cases, it may be the person's way of getting attention, but surely this person has deep psychological problems and needs mental counseling to deal with such problems. Always let an expert deal with threats of suicide.

▶ DEALING WITH LONELINESS

You probably think of the older, lonely person as one who lives alone in the heart of the city in a tiny apartment with no contact with friends and loved ones. However, even though your patient now lives in your home and is surrounded by loved ones, loneliness can still be a problem. Your patient may fear isolation, especially if he is unable to go out of the house. He needs contact with friends and persons his own age. A telephone in the patient's room can provide contact with friends. You and your family will also be a great help in preventing loneliness. Provide diversional activities and encourage other family members outside the home to visit him to relieve his boredom.

If your patient complains of loneliness, he may actually be saying more. Perhaps he is saying, "I need love," or "I need to be touched." Your patient's spouse is probably deceased, and he no longer enjoys the intimacies of sex or merely cuddling or holding another person. The act of a simple touch can do much to say to your patient, "You're still wanted, and we do love you." Simply sitting and holding the patient's hand while you talk with him or touching his shoulder as you walk by could do more for his morale than your actual conversation. Some families demonstrate affections openly with plenty of hugging and kissing while others do not. Perhaps you have never been openly affectionate to your patient, or he to you, but at least offer your hand and notice his response. The patient may greedily grab for your touch, or he may push it away; take your cue from his response.

▶ SEXUAL FEELINGS OF THE ELDERLY

Although sexual activity diminishes with age, many older adults still desire and engage in sexual activity. Medications, menopause, bodily changes due to illness, and a change in body image all contribute to decreased sexual desire and impotence. Discuss these problems with your physician. The person who has led an active sex life will probably continue to engage in sexual activities even in old age.

> Mr. T., a widower, is 79 years old and has resided with his daughter for the last year after suffering from a fractured hip. Mr. T. is active in the local senior citizens center and has become friends with a widow near his age. Mr. T.'s daughter was happy that her father had made friends with the woman until one day he asked his daughter to drive him to his "lady friend's" home so that they could be alone together.
>
> His daughter's first response was, "Dad, do you want people to call you a 'dirty old man'? Does this woman have no shame?" An argument followed. Embarrassed and angry, Mr. T. spent the next few days in his room and refused to go to the center.
>
> Finally, Mr. T.'s daughter talked with a social worker at the center. She learned that her father's feelings were normal (whether companionship of the opposite sex, hand holding, cuddling, or actual sexual intercourse). Eventually, she not only drove her father to his "lady friend's" home, but she also invited the lady to their home and gave them privacy in her father's room. Mr. T. has been happy in this relationship. Although it took his daughter a little time to accept it, she learned that sexual feelings are normal regardless of age.

▶ DEALING WITH ANXIETY

Anxiety is another common problem among the elderly. The older person may feel anxious about the new living arrangements, and his illness will be a constant source of anxiety. If you or your family are anxious, this anxiety will be felt by your patient. Try to keep your home atmosphere fairly quiet. The older person who has lived in a quiet home for years will become anxious in a home with blaring music, door slamming, and loud voices.

Try to discover the cause of your patient's anxiety. Sometimes the causes might sound petty to you. For example, a man could be worried about the roof of his former home leaking. To you this will sound like a poor reason to worry because the patient no longer lives in that home. But to your patient it is a real worry. For you to reply, "It's foolish of you to worry about that house," would only increase the anxiety. A better reply would be, "I know how much you love that old house. Do you want me to send a carpenter over to check the roof?"

Do not argue with an anxious person. This only increases anxiety. At times, you may have to report such feelings of anxiety to your physician. This is especially true if your patient is too anxious to sleep well at night. The physician will probably prescribe a mild tranquilizer (sedative) for your patient.

Also be aware that as an unwanted side effect, some medications can actually cause anxiety and nervousness. The physician should review your patient's current list of medications to rule out this possibility.

▶ DEALING WITH OTHER EMOTIONS

Feelings of despair, hopelessness, and loss are also common among the elderly. Your patient might express these feelings by stating, "Why is God punishing me? Why am I so sick?" Indeed, these are difficult questions to answer. Your best response would be to ask a question that would enable the patient to talk about these feelings. You can reply, "You seem angry (or depressed) about your illness. I can understand that. Are you feeling worse today?"

All individuals, no matter what age, resort to styles of behavior to help them cope with their situation. For instance, an ill person might refuse to take medications because taking medications would mean that he is actually sick. Your best response could be, "Your medicine is to keep you well. Dr. Harvey ordered this medicine because he wants you to stay well, and I want you to stay well."

Some elderly persons become deeply involved with politics. Sometimes, to their way of thinking, their illness is directly related to the Democratic or Republican party or perhaps the president. This behavior of transferring the cause of illness to someone else is this person's way of coping with his illness.

Regression is a common form of behavior. The person is unable to face his illness or situation, so he retreats to childish or childlike behavior such as throwing a temper tantrum. Anger or tantrums may occur because you have asked your patient to perform a task which he knows he is incapable of performing. We all express our anger at times, and if your patient is going through a particularly trying period, you can understand the reason for his anger. You should remain calm. Your reaction to this anger is important, and how you react could well determine whether there will be further outbursts of anger. You could say, "You're angry right now. We'll discuss this later when you've calmed down."

Those suffering with senility sometimes have no control over their behavior and cannot help their angry outbursts. However, if your patient is not senile and his outbursts become frequent, you may have to employ other measures. If you are unable to discover the reason for these outbursts, consult your physician; a mental health evaluation might be recommended.

If your patient's outbursts begin to affect you and other family members, it is time to call your patient and immediate family together for a meeting to discuss this problem. You will have to frankly inform your patient that you cannot accept such behavior and that he is not conforming to the rules previously agreed upon.

Reminiscing

All of us like to reminisce or recall past events from time to time, but as a person grows old, he tends to do this more frequently. The older person living in your home may love to sit for hours and tell of past experiences and events. This is a normal process, and it is believed that reminiscing is an older person's way of accepting that the end of his life is nearing. Looking through photograph albums, old letters, and cards will all bring back memories for your patient. Reminiscing about the past will give him a review of his life, and he may decide, "Yes, my life has been good."

On the other hand, if reminiscing stirs up old problems that were never resolved or feelings of guilt, your patient's conclusion may be, "My life was not successful." In this instance, you might be able to help him work through some of his past failures and disappointments.

▶ SENILITY (SENILE DEMENTIA)

Certain changes that occur in the elderly are classified as senile changes. Senile dementia takes in a wide range of diseases including Alzheimer's disease, Multi-infarct Dementia, and Pick's disease. Symptoms of these illnesses may include mental confusion, a decreased memory, a decreased attention span, and difficulty adjusting to or recognizing surroundings. These changes are related to specific changes in the brain, damage to an actual area of brain tissue, changes in the circulation of the brain, or atrophy or shrinking of brain tissue.

It is sometimes difficult for physicians to differentiate between the many types of dementia, and sometimes only an autopsy after death can provide an accurate diagnosis. For example, plaques and tangles are found in the brain of patients suffering from Alzheimer's disease when an autopsy is performed after death.

The symptoms of dementia can be deceiving. Drugs, depression, chemical imbalances, or even sight and hearing losses can cause symptoms similar to dementia, and these conditions are all reversible. A complete medical checkup, including a neurological examination, is important to discover if any of these problems are causing the symptoms of dementia. Senile dementia, or becomimg senile, was once thought to be part of the normal process of growing old, but it is now recognized as an illness.

Not all elderly become senile or suffer from dementia, while others may exhibit these symptoms in their 50s or 60s. Forgetting one appointment does not mean a person is senile. Some elderly persons in their 90s show no symptoms of senility.

There is no cure for senile dementia. There are no symptom relieving medications, although antidepressants are sometimes ordered to help combat depression and tranquilizers to ease anxiety. It is believed that the progress of dementia can be slowed if the patient is kept as physically and mentally active as possible.

Some older persons may have difficulty recognizing their surroundings during the night or when they first awaken in the morning, and it is thought that this is because the circulation of the brain has slowed during sleep. This may not be a problem after a daytime nap.

The degree of your patient's dementia will govern the type of care you administer. It is important to provide a safe environment: avoid using scatter rugs; use a bed that is low to the floor; have your patient's room downstairs—if possible—to prevent use of stairs; do not change the position of the furniture. Establish a schedule for your patient. Be consistent. There should be a set time for eating, bathing, resting, bowel and bladder elimination, and sleeping.

Your patient's movements may be slow and awkward, but never hurry him since this will only cause more confusion and could cause an accident or fall. Senility may cause your patient to forget to dress properly. The female may put on a dress and then place her slip on top. Encourage your patient to dress himself, and if clothing needs adjusted, do this in a matter of fact, subtle way without drawing special attention to the error. Some patients suffering with senile dementia will insist upon wearing many layers of clothing, for example, several dresses and several sweaters. The layers of clothing represent security for this person.

Avoid raising your voice to talk with the senile person; he is not deaf. If the patient leaves a sentence unfinished in conversations, do not finish it for him. Of course, you will not want to take on a superior, bossy attitude.

The senile person may have some oddities of behavior due to his condition. He may want or insist upon wearing a certain item of clothing, such as a cap or sweater at all times. He may hoard certain items that you consider worthless. He may be afraid of being left alone.

The senile person should be permitted to wear the cap or sweater he so highly values. However, this item will eventually become soiled, and you can try to convince him it should be cleaned, perhaps suggesting that he help you put it in the washing machine. If he refuses, your only alternative is to launder the cap or sweater while the patient is bathing or asleep for the night. You cannot be expected to allow the person to hoard boxes and boxes full of trinkets that range from empty hamburger cartons to old beach pebbles, but save the items that seem most important to him. If possible, store all of these treasured items in the basement or attic, but keep the patient's room as clutter free as possible to avoid accidents. From time to time you can bring a box of his collectibles to the room for him to look through.

Mental Confusion

"Every morning when I wake up I wonder what year she'll be living in." This statement was made by a daughter who cares for her mother in her home. It expresses the most devastating and painful experience you may ever have to deal with: watching someone you love suffer with mental confusion. No one can know for sure exactly what the confused person is seeing, hearing, feeling, or thinking, but surely the effects must be shattering to this person who was once a productive individual.

You may wonder why your confused patient clings to you, follows you through the house, and will not let you out of his sight. Your patient considers you his "lifeline." You are the one he depends on to function, and when you are out of sight, the patient feels he cannot function. With you he feels secure. You help bridge the gap between the real world and his world of confusion. Without you the patient may feel abandoned and helpless.

Of course, you cannot be expected to spend every minute of the day with your patient, but you can help him feel more secure when you have to leave. For example, the person who fears being alone would benefit from the use of an intercom system to keep in touch with you in other rooms of the house. These are available at a local electronics dealer. Announce your whereabouts often, and just drop by your patient's room from time to time to ask if he needs anything.

Although the confused person has a poor concept of time, you could make him feel more secure by providing some idea when you will return. For example, if the patient watches television, you might say, "When the noon news show is on, I'll be here to get your lunch." Or you could say, "I'll be back to see you before Alice (your daughter) comes home from school."

Leaving your patient in the care of another person may be difficult at first. When employing the help of someone outside your home to care for your patient, consider this person's past experience with confused individuals and ask for references. To help your patient and new companion become more acquainted, you will want to be present the first few times the two are together. In this way, you can observe your patient's response to this companion and the companion's response to your patient. Your patient will feel more secure with a new companion if you do not abruptly thrust this person on him and then leave. Refrain from calling this person a sitter or baby sitter. Companion or helper is better.

After caring for your confused patient for a time, you will probably notice that at certain times of the day he seems more alert. By late afternoon or evening, he may become more confused and restless. If possible, plan to spend more time with your patient during these periods. The physician may prescribe a tranquilizer if your patient is severely restless or anxious, and giving this medication just prior to this may be helpful. Also provide a quiet environment during times of greater confusion and restlessness.

Bath time is usually distressing for a confused person as taking a bath makes many demands on your patient. He must remove the "secure" clothing from his body and expose his nudity to you. He might actually fear the water or not recognize the bathtub or shower as a bathtub or a shower. To make your patient feel more secure, your behavior should be matter of fact and consistent. Tell him you are removing his slacks as you remove them. If your patient can undress himself, you might have to help by giving simple instructions, such as, "Unbutton your shirt now," touching the button as you speak.

At times, your patient may not recognize you or his surroundings. This will be painful to you, but how frightening it must be to the patient. You might have to remind him several times a day who you are or where he is. Simply say, "I'm Connie, your daughter. This is your room and this is your bed."

Your patient may actually suffer from hallucinations. One elderly man who held a top executive position during his working years, told his wife he saw striking workers out in the yard each evening. Arguing that there were no strikers only made him angry, but it helped if his wife walked him outside to show him there really were no strikers. Another man frequently heard voices that he believed were the voices of spies.

Wandering. If your patient tends to wander about during the night, consider applying side rails to the bed. Be sure, however, to explain why you are doing this, and be ready to help him to the bathroom if you hear him moving about in bed. Some patients will attempt to climb out over the side rails. If your patient usually becomes restless at 2 A.M., awaken him at 1:30 to assist him to the bathroom.

Wandering habits can sometimes be dangerous. If your patient tends to wander from the house, you will have to keep all the doors locked. The wandering patient should wear an identification bracelet. Gates, such as those used for babies, can be used at doorways indoors. Wandering might seem like an aimless, restless motion to you, and it is difficult to say why a confused person wanders. But perhaps he does have a goal in mind. Perhaps he is looking for the bathroom, going to the store, or trying to find his former home.

If your patient's dementia is not severe, you will probably be able to take him on outings, and you should encourage him to be active outside the home as long as possible. For the patient with severe dementia, you may have to schedule outings, such as doctor's appointments, at the time of day he is best able to cope with stress.

Physical condition permitting, give your patient small chores such as dusting, folding laundry, or washing dishes. Even though the patient may refold the same stack of laundry for hours, you should praise all efforts. He likes to have something to do to help pass the time. Other diversions include listening to music, listening to the radio, and working jigsaw puzzles. Sometimes just holding an object in his hands is helpful to occupy the time. This could be a small box of trinkets, a heavy string of wooden beads, or a few playing cards. Exercise is important. Walking, dancing, and exercising to music may be enjoyed by your patient.

Rules for Caring for the Confused Patient. Here are some suggestions to help you relate to and care for your confused patient.

1. Assure that your patient's physical condition is cared for as much as possible. Have vision and hearing evaluated. He should wear his hearing aid and eye glasses.
2. Keep the environment safe.
3. Keep the atmosphere relaxed.
4. Never hurry your patient.
5. Do not talk about, or in front of, your senile patient as if he were not there.
6. Use short, simple sentences and instructions.

7. Wait for your patient's reply.
8. Be calm and consistent in your behavior.
9. At times you may have to be firm, but do it calmly.
10. Do not ridicule or tease.
11. Encourage exercise and activity.
12. Humor can and should be used, but laugh *with* your patient, not *at* him.

Keeping Your Patient in Touch. Even though your patient is mentally confused, whether this be to a slight or severe degree, there are ways you can help the patient be more aware of his surroundings. Think of yourself; there have probably been times when you lost track of time. Perhaps one day while busy with daily chores, you realized you were unsure whether it was Wednesday or Thursday. To a confused person, time and days slip by unnoticed. Sometimes a night's sleep is followed by a routine day, by one nap and then another, and your patient loses touch with time.

To help keep your patient oriented to time, hang a large calendar in his room. Every day during your bathing routine or while having your morning break together, call attention to the calendar. State the day of the week, numerical date, month, and year. If possible, have your patient repeat this, and then mark off the date with a marker. Your discussion could proceed in this way: "Today is Wednesday the 18th of November. The year is 1987. In two weeks it will be Thanksgiving." Your patient can then mark off the date and repeat what you have said.

Try to break up your patient's routine by planning special days. Perhaps attending church on Sunday, a shopping trip on Friday, or going to visit friends on a special day of the week would be enjoyable.

Also try to keep your patient in touch with current events. Spend a few minutes each night going through the newspaper with your patient. Many confused patients have no idea who is the current president of the United States. You do not have to go into great detail about current news—just skim a few headlines if that is all the patient's attention span will allow.

It is true that what we learn first is the most easily retained, while what is learned last is most easily lost. This is why if your patient is confused, he might not know the name of the town he is presently living in but can vividly describe the town, street, and street number of a home lived in 40 years ago. Reminiscence therapy is a fairly new technique in which the confused person reviews events of the past. Photograph albums will be very helpful for this technique. Put yourself in your confused loved one's place; you cannot remember where you are or what year it is, but you can recognize a photograph of Uncle Harry back in 1942. What a relief this must be for the confused person. He is able to remember something. His world is not totally blurred.

It is not unusual for a confused 85-year-old woman to begin speaking about her mother as if she were still alive. She might say, "When Mother comes, I'm going to go home with her." Gently, your reply can be, "Annie, you're 85 years old. If your mother were still alive she would have to be at least 105 years old." At times this response does seem to spark reasoning in the confused person's mind, and she might reply, "You're right. My mother couldn't be alive."

Do not be disappointed, however, if this is not the response. If Annie insists that her mother is still alive, avoid arguing with her. Perhaps in a few days you can try the reply once more. Arguing with a confused person only causes him to become angry and more insistent. Teasing, joking, or playing tricks on a confused person only frustrates him. Therefore, never ridicule, tease, or argue with the senile person.

Above all, a senile person, despite appearance, behavior, and oddities, is an individual who deserves respect. The person suffering with senile dementia is not "crazy" or mentally ill. If you do not enjoy being with and caring for a senile person, do not invite this person to live in your home. Your feelings will be conveyed to your patient. More than anything he needs physical comfort, a simple life, understanding, and love.

Alzheimer's Disease

Alzheimer's disease is thought to be the most common type of senile dementia. The disease begins slowly, and the patient's symptoms may not be noticed until they become more severe. Perhaps only then will the family look back and say they had noticed occasional memory loss and vagueness several years before. The course of the disease may run from five to fifteen years.

As Alzheimer's advances, the patient needs assistance with personal hygiene, memory loss is obvious, and he is disoriented to time. During the last stage, the patient suffers severe memory loss and severe disorientation. Mood and personality changes occur. Activities of daily living, such as eating, dressing, and toileting, become a problem. Speech becomes incoherent.

Although the cause of Alzheimer's disease is still unknown, many theories exist. Hereditary factors are believed to play a role in some cases, but isolated cases in which the disease has not occurred in any past generation can also be found. Abnormally high protein levels, chemical imbalances, and trace metals are found in the brain of the patient, but it is not clear if these findings are a result of the disease or the cause.

Parkinson's Disease

Parkinson's disease is a disease of the central nervous system which affects the brain centers controlling movement. The most easily recognized symptom is tremors or shaking of the hands and body. Other symptoms include a slowness of movement with a bent posture, muscle rigidity, a masklike facial expression, difficulty swallowing, depression, and speech problems. Severe symptoms of senile dementia occur in advanced cases. This disease rarely strikes before the age of 60, and although it is progressive, its symptoms can be relieved with medications.

▶ CASE HISTORIES

This chapter has dealt with physical and emotional factors you may encounter in caring for an elderly patient. Consider three case studies of such patients.

Case History Number One

Mrs. M. is 85 years old. She suffers from congestive heart failure, is incontinent of urine, and must wear diapers. She walks only short distances with a walker. Mrs. M. resides with her 60-year-old daughter and her daughter's husband. Her room is located in a downstairs room of the house, and an inexpensive intercom is connected to her daughter's upstairs bedroom. Mrs. M. uses nasal oxygen during the night.

Although she has limited mobility, Mrs. M. enjoys being in the kitchen and helping her daughter with the cooking. She has many prized recipes she loves to copy and share with friends and visitors.

Mrs. M.'s son-in-law built ramps for easier mobility of her wheelchair, and she enjoys sitting on the screened porch on summer days. It is fairly difficult for Mrs. M.'s family to place her in the car, but weather permitting, each Saturday they help her into the car (along with her portable oxygen tank in case of an emergency) and take a leisurely drive, eventually arriving at a local fast-food restaurant. Because getting her in and out of the car is difficult, the family eats in the car. Mrs. M. usually orders a plain hamburger, french fries without salt (most fast-food chains will comply with this request), and a milk shake.

Although this does not sound like much of an outing, it is a very special day for Mrs. M., one she looks forward to all week.

Case History Number Two

Mrs. T. is 75 years old and although in good physical health, she suffers from senility. She resides with her daughter and her family. Mrs. T. used to speak constantly of her own children as if they were infants, and she often aroused her daughter in the middle of the night to tell her one of her babies was crying. One day one of Mrs. T.'s teenage grandchildren noticed a stray cat outside and brought it in to give it a saucer of milk. Mrs. T. was instantly engrossed with the cat. Now she sees that the cat is properly fed. The cat has a bed to sleep in right outside of Mrs. T.'s bedroom, and she spends hours holding, petting, grooming, and talking to her cat. Mrs. T. still suffers from periods of confusion, but her condition has improved since she has her cat, Susie, to care for.

Case History Number Three

Mr. G. is 78 years old. He has resided with his son and daughter-in-law for the past ten years. Mr. G. was in good health until he had a severe heart attack. Upon his return from the hospital, he simply went to bed, going so far as announcing that he would be dying soon and planning every detail of his funeral. His appetite was poor, he only got out of bed to go to the bathroom, and despite all attempts of his family to motivate him, he could talk of nothing but his impending death. After two weeks of this behavior, a visiting minister mentioned a parishioner of his who had also suffered a heart attack, was ten years older than Mr. G., and now kept active at the local community center for the elderly. The parishioner began to visit Mr. G. After a time, Mr. G.'s condition improved. The two men became friends, and eventually Mr. G. also joined in the activities at the community center.

CHAPTER 11

SPECIAL PROCEDURES

▶ USING AND ADMINISTERING OXYGEN

As the primary caregiver for your patient, you may be called upon to administer oxygen.

Oxygen is a colorless, odorless, and tasteless gas which is essential to life. The air around us is made up of 21 percent oxygen. The supplemental oxygen that is prescribed by a physician is almost 100 percent medically pure, thus it is considered a medication.

If your patient is to use oxygen at home, it is probably in the form of an oxygen concentrator (a machine which makes its own oxygen from the air), liquid oxygen in a cylinder, or tank oxygen. Small tanks of oxygen are available for emergencies or when it is impossible to use oxygen from another source, for example, when riding in an automobile or during a power failure.

Oxygen is measured in liters per minute. If oxygen is ordered for your patient, following the directions exactly is important. Set the flow meter at the prescribed liters per minute and use it for the specified amount of time. Using more oxygen than prescribed could cause severe respiratory complications. If a little is good, receiving more is definitely not better.

Oxygen Safety Rules

Oxygen does support combustion. This means that anything present in an oxygen enriched atmosphere will burn faster. To prevent a fire, follow these rules.

1. DO NOT allow open flames or burning tobacco in the room where oxygen is being used. Place NO SMOKING signs in the room where oxygen is being used as reminders for visitors.
2. DO NOT use electric razors, heaters, or any other electrical equipment in an oxygen enriched atmosphere.
3. DO NOT cover oxygen equipment or tubing with any type of material.
4. DO NOT oil or grease equipment.
5. DO NOT use aerosol sprays in the vicinity of oxygen.
6. Turn off the oxygen completely when not in use.
7. DO NOT store oxygen in a confined area.
8. DO NOT store oxygen near sources of heat, such as radiators, heat ducts, or steam pipes.
9. Avoid using nylon clothing or woolen blankets which could produce sparks.
10. DO NOT attempt to repair or adjust the equipment your-self—call your supplier for trained help.
11. Check all tubing and humidifier connections for leaks and kinks.
12. Check the flow liter meter at intervals and keep it at the prescribed dosage.

The Patient Using Oxygen

Oxygen can be given to the patient in many forms, such as intermittent positive pressure or by mask. Although once commonly used, oxygen tents are rarely used today. Nasal oxygen is a common form currently used. A small tubing (nasal cannula) is attached to the patient's face by securing the tubing over the ears and placing a small prong into each nostril. If your patient is using nasal oxygen, encourage him to breathe through the nose with his mouth closed. (See Figure 1.)

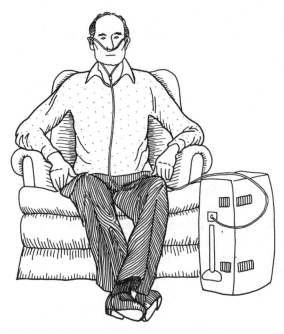

Figure 1. A patient using nasal oxygen.

Some patients complain that their "nose runs" more frequently while using oxygen, and you must keep the nasal area dry in order to prevent irritation. Apply a water soluble lubricant to this area. The tubing over the ears sometimes causes irritation also, and small pieces of soft flannel or cotton can be placed at these areas.

Oxygen is a dry gas, so in order to make it more humid, it is passed through a humidifier before it reaches the patient. The simplest form of humidifier is the bubble humidifier, a container of distilled water on the oxygen concentrator machine. You will be instructed to keep the water at a certain level in the bubble humidifier.

The oxygen supplier will provide enough tubing to allow your patient to walk short distances while using oxygen. Use care to prevent tripping over the oxygen lines or getting them tangled with furniture.

The physician may routinely order blood gases to be drawn to determine the level of oxygen in your patient's blood. This blood is drawn from an artery (as opposed to most blood being drawn from a vein), and a trained person, usually a respiratory therapist, will perform this procedure.

If oxygen is ordered for your patient, note in your diary the flow rate (liters per minute), the amount of time it is to be used, and the name and telephone number of your supplier. Your supplier will have an emergency number which you can call 24 hours a day in the event of an emergency. Do not hesitate to call this number if you are having a problem with oxygen equipment.

The Patient with Emphysema

Emphysema, sometimes known as Chronic Obstructive Lung Disease (COLD) or Chronic Obstructive Pulmonary Disease (COPD), is a destructive lung disease. Usually the disease has occurred for many years before obvious symptoms of shortness of breath become noticeable. Smoking and air pollution are the major causes of emphysema. Basically, with emphysema the tiny air sacs of the lungs lose their elasticity. There is increased mucus secretions and narrowing of the airways. A "barrel-shaped" chest is commonly seen in the person suffering with emphysema. Chronic coughing, wheezing, and increased shortness of breath become more severe as the disease advances. The patient tires easily, and breathing becomes hard work.

Treatment includes the use of medications which help dilate the airways and loosen secretions. The patient with emphysema is prone to lung infections, and antibiotics are given at the first sign of infection because repeated infection causes even more lung damage. Oxygen therapy is used in advanced cases.

▶ Caring for a New Incision

If your patient has recently had surgery, you may be a little timid about caring for the fresh incision. However, your surgeon will give you specific instructions about cleaning and inspecting this area. Ask for these instructions in writing so you can refer to them as necessary.

Dressings are not used as frequently to cover new incisions as they once were, so the incision may not have a dressing. The sutures (stitches) or wire clamps or staples may still be in place. At times the surgeon places special strips of adhesive directly over the incision to help hold the edges together. These special strips should not be removed. Some of these adhesive strips will eventually fall off. Consult the surgeon about this, so you will not be alarmed if it occurs.

Keep the incisional area clean and dry. If it does become soiled, such as by urine or bowel movement, gently cleanse it with mild soap and water and gently pat dry. Inspect the incision area for signs of redness, swelling, or discharge. Ask your physician about bathing. Most patients are now permitted to take showers as soon as their condition permits. Do not apply salves, lotions, or ointments to the incision unless instructed to do so. Return to the physician at the designated time to have sutures removed.

If your patient does have a dressing, be certain you understand all instructions about caring for the incision and dressing. The dressing is usually changed at least daily, or more often if there is a large amount of drainage present or it becomes wet or soiled. Packaged sterile dressings are available at the pharmacy in assorted types and sizes.

Always wash your hands before and after caring for the dressing, and have your work area as clean as possible. Disposable gloves may be worn if you prefer. Gently remove the old dressing. If it sticks to the wound, moisten the outside of the dressing with sterile water (water that has been boiled for ten minutes and then cooled). Discard the old dressing in a plastic bag after first noting the type and amount of drainage.

Inspect the incisional area for any signs of redness, swelling, pus, or odor. If you have been instructed to clean the incision, use a sterile gauze dressing. Gather the sterile dressing in your fingertips by grasping the back outer edges at the corners. Holding it in this manner will provide a sterile inner surface to use during cleansing. Use the cleaning solution that is ordered. If sterile water is ordered, your home health nurse will supply it, or it can be purchased at a pharmacy. Wet the gauze dressing with the solution and cleanse from top to bottom of the incision line. Use gentle pressure and do not rub. Use one stroke and do not go back over the area with the same gauze dressing. Instead, use another moistened dressing and repeat this step if the incisional area needs further cleansing. Do not try to remove any crusted (scabbed) tissue if present. This will eventually fall off during the normal healing process. Use as many gauze dressings as necessary to cleanse the area, then use another dry dressing to gently dry the area.

Now you are ready to apply a dry sterile dressing. Do not touch the part of the dressing that will come in contact with the incision. Peel open the dressing package, exposing the entire dressing. Lay it on a flat surface in its opened package and remove it by grasping an outer back corner. Lay the dressing over the incision and secure it with adhesive tape. A paper adhesive tape is best for patients with delicate skin.

If a dressing is ordered to be changed by complete sterile technique, the home health nurse will do this or instruct you on the procedure.

Observe the incision for signs of inflammation or infection, such as redness, pain, or swelling. An incision that has been healing well and suddenly begins to ooze any type of drainage, clear or containing pus or blood, should be reported to your physician immediately. Generalized symptoms may also indicate infection of an incision. Report any elevation in temperature, headache, nausea, loss of appetite, or chills.

Sometimes it is very difficult to remove the residue of adhesive tape from the skin. Special products are available to remove old tape marks. Baby oil may help loosen this residue, too. Use care not to get these products directly on the incision, and follow the directions carefully.

▶ COLLECTING SPECIMENS

Collecting a Urine Specimen

Your physician may ask you to collect a urine specimen from your patient.

Some controversy exists about whether it is best to obtain the first voided specimen in the morning or the second. Follow your doctor's preference about this. Because some components in the urine will break down within two hours, if you are expected to take a urine specimen for a doctor's appointment at three in the afternoon, it is best to get the specimen about an hour before appointment time.

The physician may provide a special container in which to collect the specimen, or you may use a small, clean jar. The jar and lid may be boiled in water for about ten minutes to assure its cleanliness. The laboratory will need at least one ounce of urine (about three large tablespoonsful). Try to collect about four ounces of urine.

A good time to collect the urine specimen is directly after a bath when the genital area is very clean. If this is not possible, have your patient wash the genital area well with soap and water, rinsing and drying well. If your patient is unable to perform this alone, you will have to wash the area. To collect the specimen, the patient starts the urinary flow into the commode, and after a few seconds catches the amount for the urine specimen in the container. This is called a clean catch, midstream urine specimen and is used because it is best to catch the urine after some has passed through the urinary opening, and flushing the area of bacteria. Seal the container immediately after collecting the specimen, being careful not to touch the interior of the container which will come in contact with the urine.

If your patient is unable to void in the commode or bedside commode, collect the specimen in a urinal for a male or a bedpan for a female. Clean the urinal or bedpan well with soap and water, and scald it with very hot water before collecting the specimen. As always, wash your hands before and after this procedure.

A urinalysis is the usual test performed on urine. A urinalysis gives your physician much information, such as the dilution of urine, whether it is acid or alkaline, and the presence of abnormal cells (blood cells, yeast, or bacteria).

Another common urine test is a culture and sensitivity (C and S). For this test the urine must be as clean as possible. A special cleaning solution is used to cleanse the genital area. To collect this specimen from a male, the urinary opening and penis are cleansed with this solution. He then voids, catching the midstream urine in a sterile container. Obtaining this specimen from a female patient is more difficult because the close proximity with the vagina may allow vaginal secretions to come in contact with the urine. The labia and area around the urinary opening are cleansed with the special solution, and the midstream urine is collected.

A culture and sensitivity is done to determine whether an infection is present in the urine. It also tells the physician what antibiotics will combat this infection. Allow about three days for the results of a C and S since the bacteria must "grow" under laboratory conditions.

Collecting a Stool Specimen

Although collecting a stool specimen is not pleasant, it gives your physician much needed information. It is used to determine the presence of blood in the stool (this may be blood cells that are only seen by use of a microscope) and the presence of parasites such as pinworms. Have your patient use a clean bedpan to pass a bowel movement. Then using a tongue blade, obtain about 3/4 teaspoon of bowel movement from one area of the stool and a second specimen from another area of the stool. Place the specimens in a clean container—a small milk carton or a disposable margarine container will do. Seal the container and store it in a cool place or take it to the laboratory or physician's office as ordered.

Collecting a stool specimen is unpleasant. If the odor is very offensive to you, try saturating a cotton ball with perfume and tucking it under your collar line. In this way, you can smell the fragrance of the perfume while working. You can also use this cotton ball and perfume method while doing other offensive tasks, such as bowel care, emptying the bedpan or bedside commode, and so forth.

Small specially prepared packets are now available to analyze bowel movement, and the directions are on the package. Only a small smear of bowel movement is needed, and you may use a cotton-tipped applicator to apply the bowel movement to the special area on the packet. If your patient does not have a bowel movement daily, do not be concerned. Just collect a specimen as bowel movements occur. When each area of the packet contains a specimen, it can be mailed or taken to the physician or laboratory.

▶ FASTING FOR BLOOD WORK

If your physician orders blood tests in which it is necessary for your patient to fast prior to the drawing of the blood, it means the patient is not to have anything to eat or drink prior to the test. Your patient should begin fasting at midnight on the evening before the test. Usually all medications are held, but if your patient is taking a medication which it is imperative to take on schedule, the physician may tell you to give this medication with a small amount of water. If you are in doubt about this, consult your physician.

CHAPTER 12

SPECIAL PROBLEMS

▶ POOR VISION

If your patient has poor vision, your main goal is that he will be as independent and self-sufficient as possible. The problems of the partially seeing person are unique. This person is not necessarily considered legally blind, does not need a guide dog, and in some instances may not even wear glasses. Yet many partially seeing individuals are unable to read the newspaper or street signs.

Your patient should have regular eye examinations. If poor vision, sometimes called low vision or partially seeing, is confirmed, it will be necessary to seek the assistance of a low vision specialist. The low vision specialist can prescribe special equipment for your patient. Many devices are available for the partially seeing, such as proper lighting with special illuminators and magnifiers. However, acquiring such equipment does not simply mean increasing the wattage of the patient's reading light or buying a magnifying glass at a local department store. The patient should be encouraged to use any special equipment the low vision specialist prescribes. (These devices are discussed later in the chapter.)

If your patient does have poor vision, color and depth perception may be a problem. You are probably familiar with the practice of painting the edges of stair treads with a bright paint, such as orange or yellow, to help define the edges of steps. Try this technique in your own home, using brightly colored reflector tape.

The use of contrasting colors will also help. Perhaps your patient is very clumsy about sitting down in his chair. If the flooring and the chair are both brown, it could be that your patient has difficulty distinguishing the actual chair. You can change the color of the chair without going to the expense of having it recovered by simply placing two brightly colored bath towels over the chair, one over the back and one over the seat portion.

Use contrasting colors wherever your patient seems to be having problems distinguishing shapes and areas. Reflector tape can be used on such areas as handrails along the walls and stairs, along the edge of the bathtub, along doorways, and on the hot water faucet.

Write notes and messages with a thick, felt-tipped marker. Keep a list of emergency numbers by your telephone. Write them in large print with a felt-tipped marker to enable your patient to use them. Also reduce glare wherever it is a problem.

Common Eye Disorders of the Elderly

Presbyopia is a common eye disorder called the sight of aging. It refers to difficulties in near seeing caused by gradual reduction in strength of accommodation (ability to focus for near). Persons generally develop this problem in their 40s, 50s, or 60s. As a person loses ability to change focus from distant to near, he can be helped by magnifying (convex) glasses.

Another common eye disorder is glaucoma, a disease characterized by increased pressure within the eye, often because of defects in the drainage mechanism through which the aqueous fluid flows out of the eye. Since the fluid tends to be formed continuously, the pressure builds up. If the increased pressure is not relieved, the eye will be damaged. Glaucoma can occur at any age, but it is most common over age 40. Early detection is important. Usually the person suffering with glaucoma does not realize there is a visual problem. He can read an eye chart, yet the side vision is slowly closing in, and a condition called tunnel vision results. This vision resembles looking through a long train tunnel. Most cases can be kept under control with medication and/or surgery.

Cataracts are a clouding in the normally clear lens of the eye. The rate of progression of cataracts varies from person to person, often between the two eyes of the same person. Resting the eyes will not prevent the development of cataracts, nor will use of the eyes cause them. The most common cataract is the senile cataract which comes with advancing years. With age, just as the cells of the elderly person's skin become thicker, the normally transparent cells of the lens of the eye also become denser, causing a cataract to develop. Surgery is the only currently recognized treatment.

Other common eye problems of the elderly include retinal disease and macular degeneration. Prompt diagnosis and treatment are essential to prevent further eye damage and possible blindness.

If your patient has an abrupt change in vision, throbbing or pain in the eye, a reduced field of vision, unusual blurring, double vision, or blood spots on the front of the eye, seek immediate medical attention.

Low Vision Aids[7]

Many devices are available to help the person with low or poor vision, but first the person has to accept the fact that he has low vision. The person also has to have some useful visual field or some useful central vision, along with a strong desire to see better. It will take time and effort to learn to use the various visual aids which are available. The medical condition causing the visual problem should receive appropriate attention from an opthalmologist, a medical doctor specializing in the treatment and surgery of the eyes.

Low vision equipment falls into three categories.

1. Nonoptical aids and approach magnification includes the control of illumination (light) and contrast, or bringing things closer, such as sitting closer to the television, special lamps, filters, and large print.

2. Optical aids control focus, image clarity, or magnification. These include hand or stand magnifiers, head borne magnifiers, contact lenses, and telescopes.

3. Electronic aids often combine the elements of the other two principles. These include illuminated magnifiers and closed circuit televisions (video magnifiers).

Other aids now available for the person with low vision include high intensity magnifying lamps; novels, cookbooks, and crossword puzzle books in large print; talking desktop alarm clocks; digital alarm clocks with 1 3/4 inch numbers; low vision wrist watches; templates for check-writing guides, signature guides, and envelope-addressing guides; playing cards with extra large numbers; and talking bath scales. These aids and many others along with much useful information can be obtained for the person with poor or low vision by writing to:

National Association for Visually Handicapped
22 West 21st Street, 6th Floor
New York, NY 10010

The National Library Service for the Blind and Physically Handicapped works through local and regional libraries to provide free library service to persons unable to read or use standard printed materials because of a visual or physical impairment. It provides information on blindness and physical handicaps on request. For more information write to:

National Library Service for the Blind and
Physically Handicapped
Library of Congress,
Washington, D.C. 20542
or telephone 800-424-9100

▶ POOR HEARING

Hearing impairment becomes more common after the age of 65. Loss of hearing due to the aging process is called presbycusis, and the degree in loss of hearing may vary from slight to severe. Some older persons may not suffer from hearing loss, but they may appear to be hard of hearing because they are unable to understand what is being said. This condition is caused by hardening of the arteries in the brain, and it will not be helped by a hearing aid. Speak slowly and distinctly to this person; shouting is unnecessary. Repeat your words as necessary, and use short, simple sentences.

Types of Hearing Loss

There are two types of hearing loss: conductive and sensorineural. Conductive hearing loss is caused when an injury or disease interferes with the normal conduction of sound waves through the outer and middle ear to the inner ear. Impacted wax in the ear is one of the causes of this condition. Other causes may be more complicated.

Sensorineural hearing loss (nerve deafness) is the second type of hearing impairment. This condition may be caused by a malfunction in the inner ear, the auditory nerve or auditory center located in the brain. It is sometimes difficult for persons suffering with this condition to understand what is being said; therefore, a hearing aid may only help to a limited degree.

Some persons suffer from a mixed type of hearing loss. This is a combination of both conductive and sensorineural impairments.

Whatever your patient's hearing problem, it is important to seek the help of an audiologist, a professional trained in the treatment of hearing impairments. Refer to the telephone directory for audiologists in your area, or ask your local speech and hearing association. Usually an audiologist must be certified, and in some states a license is also required.

Hearing Aids

If your patient suffers from a condition that can be helped by a hearing aid, you will have to convince him that he actually needs a hearing aid. Having to continually shout at a person to communicate is frustrating, yet many older persons do not want to admit they actually have a hearing loss. In addition, wearing a hearing aid requires some adjustment. Encourage your patient to wear his hearing aid. Make sure it is in proper working order, and fits properly without being uncomfortable. Clean the hearing aid as instructed.

Other hearing implements are available, such as earphones for televisions and special equipment for telephones. You may obtain more information about implements available by writing to:

National Association for Hearing and Speech Action
10801 Rockville Pike
Rockville, MD 20852
Toll-free consumer Helpline 800-638-8255 (voice or TDD)

Earwax

Earwax, or cerumen, is a natural secretion of the ear. In most persons the earwax works forward to the outer ear and is removed with normal washing of the outer ear canal, but in some cases the earwax becomes hard and impacted. This can cause a hearing loss. The physician can tell you if your patient's ears are embedded with wax. In no way should this be considered unclean; nor should you think that your patient practices poor personal hygiene. The old adage not to put anything smaller than your elbow in your ear still holds true. Under no circumstances should you use cotton-tipped applicators to clean the ear because this only helps to push and pack wax into the ear canal. Use no hair pins or other implements in the ear.

Only instill ear medication and drops that are recommended by your physician since the instillation of some home remedies may cause further damage by keeping the ear moist and encouraging the growth of bacteria.

Earwax can be removed by your physician by irrigating the ear. (Usually a product to help soften the wax is used prior to irrigation.) Ear irrigation should only be performed by a physician, audiologist, or a trained nurse.

▶ CANCER

Cancer is a general term used to describe an abnormal cell growth (tumor) in the body. Some tumors are benign (not cancerous), while others are malignant. A malignant, cancerous tumor invades surrounding tissue and can spread to other regions of the body. Much medical progress has been made in the treatment of cancer. Although cancer is a very serious illness, it should not necessarily be regarded as fatal. Many persons have been cured of cancer. Skin cancer is the most common cancer, and it is the most easily treated and cured. Other cancers include breast cancer, lung cancer, colon cancer, leukemia, and Hodgkin's disease, to name a few.

If cancer is diagnosed in your patient, at first you, your patient, and your family may feel shocked, angry, confused, and frightened. You might deny that cancer is actually present. Seek support from your doctor. An oncologist, a physician who specialized in the treatment of cancer, will be recommended. Your clergy, friends, and cancer support groups can also help. Some patients and families have difficulty discussing this subject and expressing their feelings. Some friends may avoid you and your patient because they feel uncomfortable and "don't know what to say."

Treatment for cancer may include chemotherapy (the use of anticancer drugs), surgery, radiation, or a combination of these treatments. The physician will prescribe the treatment that is right for your patient. Avoid any "cures" that seem too good to be true. Over the years, many treatments that have no scientific support and are completely worthless have been promoted by unscrupulous persons.

Your patient should participate in normal activities, responsibilities, and relationships. Practice good health habits, including good skin care, bowel and bladder regularity, rest and exercise, and good nutrition. Nutrition may be a problem if your patient has a poor appetite or is taking some forms of chemotherapy. The cancer patient needs protein, but some foods containing protein, such as red meats, may actually have a bitter taste. Meats may taste better if served cold or at room temperature. Chicken, fish, eggs, cheeses, puddings, milk shakes, and nuts can be served.

Although not all cancer patients have pain, most fear that they will be in pain. Your physician will reassure you that pain can be controlled if it does occur, and he will select the proper medication.

For more information, contact your local cancer society listed in the telephone directory. (The toll-free cancer hotline is listed in Appendix D.)

▶ DIABETES

Diabetes mellitus (sugar diabetes) is a condition in which the body cannot use food properly. Normally, during the digestion process foods are broken down into sugar, and the pancreas secretes insulin into the bloodstream to keep the amount of sugar (glucose) at a consistent level. With diabetes, the pancreas does not secrete enough insulin, and the sugar level of the blood becomes too high. Symptoms of diabetes are increased urination, excessive thirst, weakness, fatigue, increased appetite, slow healing of a cut, pain or tingling of the hands and feet, and changes in vision.

Treatment of diabetes depends on the severity of the condition. Diabetics are treated with either a controlled diet, oral hypoglycemic medications which help stimulate insulin production, insulin injections, or a combination of these treatments. Exercise is also important for the diabetic.

The physician will prescribe the caloric diet that is right for your patient. This diet includes the basic four food groups. Meals should be given on a regular schedule, and the diabetic should not skip meals.

If your patient has to take insulin, your nurse will instruct you on the proper procedure for giving insulin, rotating sites of injection, and signs and symptoms of low blood sugar (hypoglycemia) and high blood sugar (hyperglycemia). Signs of high blood sugar include excessive urination, excessive thirst, headache, visual changes, nausea, vomiting, and abdominal pain. A low blood sugar can occur when there is too much insulin or too little sugar in the blood. This is also known as insulin shock or insulin reaction. Signs and symptoms include headache, irritability, shaking, sweating, and dizziness.

Diabetics should practice good skin care, including daily foot care. They should follow their diet carefully, lose weight if overweight, get routine blood sugar tests, and test urine for sugar routinely. Diabetics also need to wear an identification bracelet stating they are diabetic.

▶ STROKE

A stroke occurs when the blood flow to a portion of the brain is blocked. This can happen when there is a blood clot inside a blood vessel of the brain or neck, when a blood clot from another part of the body travels to the brain, when there is a decreased flow of blood to an area of the brain, or when a blood vessel ruptures within the brain. Depending on the portion of the brain affected by the stroke, the patient may become paralyzed on one side of the body, have speech problems, visual problems, poor control of bowel and bladder function, or impaired mental function.

Mini strokes or little strokes also occur. This is caused by a temporary blocking of blood to the brain tissue. The patient suffering from a mini stroke usually recovers completely, but this is a signal that a stroke may occur and medical attention is needed.

Depending on the severity of the stroke, the patient will need special care. This includes special skin care to prevent bedsores and an exercise routine to prevent stiff joints and contractures of muscles. Rehabilitation, including exercise, is started as soon after a stroke as possible.

Bathing may present a problem. The stroke victim will need assistance soaping and rinsing the washcloth. He will be able to wash his affected, or paralyzed, arm but not his unaffected arm. While helping him to dress, always start with the affected arm; that is, place the affected arm through the sleeve first, and then the unaffected. For undressing, do just the opposite. Remove the unaffected arm and then the paralyzed arm.

While eating, the stroke patient may have problems with his plate sliding away from him. A rubber suction cup gripper can be placed on the bottom of the plate to prevent sliding.

The physician, nurse, occupational therapist, and physical therapist will help you aid your patient in becoming as independent as possible. There are many stroke support clubs and groups. For more information contact your local heart association.

CHAPTER 13

DEATH AND DYING

▶ TALKING ABOUT DEATH

How you and your family deal with death and dying will be influenced by your own feelings about death. If you have always considered death a part of life, your outlook and attitude toward it will be natural and accepting. However, some have fearful feelings toward death. Some regard the process as the final ending of life. They have heard eerie tales about ghosts, hauntings, and deathbed curses, and so forth. They fear the unknown and feel uncomfortable talking about and facing death.

Examine your own feelings about death. Perhaps it is a subject you are comfortable about discussing with your family and your patient, but perhaps it is not. You may have experienced the death of an immediate family member. If so, recall and examine your feelings at that time as well as the reaction of other members of your immediate family.

Once you have come face to face with your own feelings about death, you are ready to decipher your patient's feelings and wishes about dying. Some ill persons will accept death willingly while others never openly discuss the subject. Because you will want to honor any requests your patient may have regarding funeral and burial arrangements, listen closely for clues your patient may be giving you regarding wishes in this matter. Some persons will not be shy about expressing their wishes. Assure this person that you will carry out any requests to the best of your ability, providing of course, that the requests are reasonable.

One patient may state, "When I go up to the hill over town (meaning the cemetery), I want to go as quietly as possible." This is your cue to expand the subject. You could ask, "Do you mean you want a small, private funeral?" You have now given your patient the opportunity to openly discuss any phase of the dying process he wishes.

This is a good time to discuss any material possessions your patient would like to have distributed to other family members. It is not unusual for many problems regarding family keepsakes and property to arise after the death of a loved one. For instance, after the mother of several daughters had died, three daughters all claimed that their mother had promised them her diamond ring, and all justly so. In order to avoid family disputes at this time of sorrow, encourage your patient to consult an attorney and obtain a written will. (Laws will vary depending on location.)

This is also a good time to discuss such topics as artificial support systems and what medical measures your patient would want performed in the event that he is unconscious or mentally incapable of making decisions. It might be helpful for you and your loved one to review *A LIVING WILL* at this time (see Figure 1).

The person who refuses to discuss dying will be a greater challenge. If you tactfully bring up the subject of burial arrangements or another topic pertinent to death and your loved one immediately changes the subject, perhaps the patient would be more comfortable discussing this matter with his priest, minister, or rabbi.

Many persons are quite clear in expressing their wish to die at home. If your patient makes this request of you, your best response will be to promise to allow him to die at home, providing he is comfortable, in no pain, and you can cope with the physical and emotional care problems that may arise during the dying process. On the other hand, if you feel having your patient die in your home would be too emotionally painful and a frightening experience, be honest with your patient by telling him so.

You need to consider the feelings of other family members, too. Some patients will need 24-hour-a-day care for weeks or even months

My Living Will
To My Family, My Physician, My Lawyer
and All Others Whom It May Concern

Death is as much a reality as birth, growth, maturity and old age—it is the one certainty of life. If the time comes when I can no longer take part in decisions for my own future, let this statement stand as an expression of my wishes and directions, while I am still of sound mind.

If at such a time the situation should arise in which there is no reasonable expectation of my recovery from extreme physical or mental disability, I direct that I be allowed to die and not be kept alive by medications, artificial means or "heroic measures". I do, however, ask that medication be mercifully administered to me to alleviate suffering even though this may shorten my remaining life.

This statement is made after careful consideration and is in accordance with my strong convictions and beliefs. I want the wishes and directions here expressed carried out to the extent permitted by law. Insofar as they are not legally enforceable, I hope that those to whom this Will is addressed will regard themselves as morally bound by these provisions.

(Optional specific provisions to be made in this space — see other side)

DURABLE POWER OF ATTORNEY (optional)

I hereby designate _____ to serve as my attorney-in-fact for the purpose of making medical treatment decisions. This power of attorney shall remain effective in the event that I become incompetent or otherwise unable to make such decisions for myself.

Optional Notarization: Signed _____

"Sworn and subscribed to   Date _____

before me this _____ day   Witness _____

of _____, 19____."
                                                       _____
                                                                        Address

_____
            Notary Public   Witness _____
              (seal)
                                                       _____
                                                                        Address

Copies of this request have been given to _____

_____   _____

(Optional) My Living Will is registered with Concern for Dying (No. _____)

Distributed by Concern for Dying, 250 West 57th Street, New York, NY 10107 (212) 246-6962

Figure 1.   Example: *A Living Will.*

THE LIVING WILL REGISTRY

In 1983, Concern for Dying instituted the Living Will Registry, a computerized file system where you may keep an up-to-date copy of your Living Will in our New York office.

What are the benefits of joining the Living Will Registry?

- CONCERN's staff will ensure that your form is filled out correctly, assign you a Registry Number and maintain a copy of your Living Will.

- CONCERN's staff will be able to refer to *your* personal document, explain procedures and options, and provide you with the latest case law or state legislation should you, your proxy or anyone else acting on your behalf need counseling or legal guidance in implementing your Living Will.

- You will receive a permanent, credit card size plastic mini-will with your Registry number imprinted on it. The mini-will, which contains your address, CONCERN's address and a short version of the Living Will, indicates that you have already filled out a full-sized, witnessed Living Will document.

How do you join the Living Will Registry?

- Review your Living Will, making sure it is up-to-date and contains any specific provisions that you want added.

- Mail a copy of your original, signed and witnessed document along with a check for $25.00 to:

   The Living Will Registry
   Concern for Dying
   250 West 57th Street, Room 831
   New York, New York 10107

   The one-time Registry enrollment fee will cover the costs of processing and maintaining your Living Will and of issuing your new plastic mini-will.

- If you have any address changes or wish to add or delete special provisions that you have included in your Living Will, please write to the Registry so that we can keep your file up to date.

TO MAKE BEST USE OF YOUR LIVING WILL

You may wish to add specific statements to the Living Will *in the space provided for that purpose above your signature.* Possible additional provisions are:

1. "Measures of artificial life-support in the face of impending death that I specifically refuse are:
   a) Electrical or mechanical resuscitation of my heart when it has stopped beating.
   b) Nasogastric tube feeding when I am paralyzed or unable to take nourishment by mouth.
   c) Mechanical respiration when I am no longer able to sustain my own breathing.
   d) _____ "

2. "I would like to live out my last days at home rather than in a hospital if it does not jeopardize the chance of my recovery to a meaningful and sentient life or does not impose an undue burden on my family."

3. "If any of my tissues are sound and would be of value as transplants to other people, I freely give my permission for such donation."

The optional Durable Power of Attorney feature allows you to name someone else to serve as your proxy in case you are unable to communicate your wishes. Should you choose to fill in this portion of the document, you must have your signature notarized.

If you choose more than one proxy for decision-making on your behalf, please give order of priority (1, 2, 3, etc.)

Space is provided at the bottom of the Living Will for notarization should you choose to have your Living Will witnessed by a Notary Public.

REMEMBER . . .

- Sign and date your Living Will. Your two witnesses, who should not be blood relatives or beneficiaries of your property will, should also sign in the spaces provided.

- Discuss your Living Will with your doctors; if they agree with you, give them copies of your signed Living Will document for them to add to your medical file.

- Give copies of your signed Living Will to anyone who may be making decisions for you if you are unable to make them yourself.

- Look over your Living Will once a year, redate it and initial the new date to make it clear that your wishes have not changed.

For additional Living Wills, or the appropriate document in those states which have passed Living Will legislation, use coupon on reverse side.

• • •

The Concern for Dying newsletter is a quarterly publication reporting the most recent developments in the field of death and dying. It contains announcements of upcoming educational conferences, workshops and symposia, as well as reviews of current literature. The Newsletter is sent to anyone who contributes $5.00 or more annually to CONCERN FOR DYING.

☐ I would like to receive the Newsletter.
☐ I would like to enroll in the Living Will Registry

• • •

Additional materials available to contributors:

☐ Questions and Answers About the Living Will
☐ Selected articles and case histories
☐ A bibliography
☐ Information on films

Figure 1 *(Continued).* Reprinted with permission of Concern for Dying, an educational council, 250 West 57th Street, NewYork, N.Y. 10107; (212) 246-6962.

during the dying process, and perhaps your family simply cannot physically and emotionally meet this demand.

Most terminally ill patients and their families look to religious and spiritual support for comfort during the dying process. Encourage and seek the counseling of your religious leader and church at this time. Even though your patient has not been a "religious person" in the past, offer this opportunity since the patient may want to "make final peace with God."

▶ DYING AT HOME

The dying patient's attitude toward death will vary. One person will willingly accept his death, while another will completely deny the fact that he is dying. One person may wish to talk about death and "put his affairs in order," while another person will be angry at everyone— including you and your family. Some will go through phases of depression. Be supportive to your patient's emotional needs at this time no matter what the attitude. Most elderly do accept their death, although in some cases this acceptance does not occur until death is imminent.

Whether expressed or not, all dying persons wish to die gracefully, comfortably, and with respect. Your most important aim for the patient dying at home is that he die with dignity. Unless death comes suddenly, the dying patient will gradually lose control of bodily functions. He will be unable to control urine and bowel movements, lose strength and use of muscles, and become more dependent upon the caregiver. This dependence may cause embarrassment to your patient.

Always use measures to prevent embarrassment. Even though your patient may be unconscious, use care not to expose him unduly while tending to personal needs. If the patient is incontinent of bowel movement, expose only the genital area or rectal area necessary for cleansing. Although odors may be a problem, make no reference to this.

The dying patient will need the same meticulous physical care (skin care, bathing, frequent position changes, and mouth care) as you have been practicing. While performing these procedures, always tell your patient what you are about to do before you do it. Even if the patient seems to be unconscious, tell him that you are about to turn him or wash his face. Speak in your normal tone. There is no need to raise your voice while caring for the unconscious or partially unconscious patient. It is thought that the sense of hearing is acute during the dying process, and since no one can say with certainty when this sense diminishes, you should assume that your patient's hearing is intact and acute until death. Also instruct all visitors not to shout or raise their voice while speaking to your patient; however, there should be no whispering among visitors in your patient's presence.

This will be a very difficult, emotional time for both you and your immediate family. Your patient may have been a part of your home for weeks, months, or years, and you will feel much sorrow knowing that death is approaching. You can gain courage and strength in the fact that you and your family have welcomed your patient into your home and cared for him to the best of your ability.

Family members other than those of your immediate family may wish to visit the patient now. Caution visitors about your patient's condition, and set up some rules concerning length of visits, based on the patient's condition. Also restrict visiting to a few persons at a time.

Visitors can sometimes be more physically and emotionally tiring for you than actually caring for your patient. During this difficult time, family members and old friends (some of whom you may not have seen for years) want to "drop in." Abide by the visiting rules you have set up. If you are tired or busy with other chores or if your patient is comfortably resting and you do not wish to have the patient disturbed, tell visitors so.

Physically, you will want to keep your patient as comfortable as possible. Moaning or restless movements are signs of pain. Notify the physician if you feel the patient is in pain. Your physician will order medication to relieve the pain. If the patient can no longer take pills or liquid medications by mouth, the medication may be ordered to be given rectally in the form of a suppository. Also change the body position frequently and use pillows to reposition your patient to promote comfort.

Change all linens, gowns, and diapers as needed. Keep the lips moist by applying lip balms, and give frequent mouth care. Swab the mouth with cotton-tipped applicators moistened with water or a mixture of 1/2 mouthwash and 1/2 water. Specially prepared cotton applicators are available at the pharmacy to help keep the mouth moist.

Keep your patient warm. However, if he is perspiring, it is a signal that he is too warm, and you should remove some of the bed covers.

With loss of muscle control and semiconsciousness or unconsciousness also comes a difficulty in swallowing. Elevate the head of the bed to a half-sitting position to ease swallowing. Offer your patient sips of water or juice if possible, but if he chokes easily, do not continue. Instead keep the mouth moist by swabbing it with cotton applicators soaked with water, the water and mouthwash mixture, or the specially prepared swabs.

As death approaches, you may notice that your patient's skin acquires a blue tinge. The extremities may become mottled or blotchy white in appearance and be cold and clammy to the touch. The body temperature may rise. Even though your patient is unconscious, the eyes may be open. Because the normal blink reflex which helps keep the eyes moist may be gone, you will want to apply soothing eye drops to keep the eyes moist.

Avoid glare in your patient's room, but keep the room well lighted. It is believed that as the eyesight diminishes, a normal amount of light is beneficial to your patient.

You will also notice respiratory changes as death approaches. The respirations may become very rapid, and you should elevate the head of the bed to aid breathing. Oxygen may be ordered at this time. In some cases, the respirations will become sporatic and even cease for intervals. This is known as Cheyne-Stokes respirations. At first, the breathing may only cease for a few seconds, but gradually this may increase to 30 seconds or more.

Your patient may also begin to accumulate secretions (mucus or phlegm) in the mouth and throat. You can remove these secretions by using a suction machine. Have the home health nurse instruct you in the proper use of the machine, so you will feel comfortable using it.

The pulse will become weaker and feel thready. It may become either rapid or slow. At times, the radial pulse (in the wrist) may not be felt for several hours before death. The pupils will become dilated (enlarge), and the blood pressure will drop.

Many families fear that they will not know when actual death has occurred, but you will know. Just sit quietly with your patient and monitor respirations. Be calm. There is no need to be frightened, and there is no rush. Dying occurs when the respirations and heartbeat have ceased for several minutes. If you wish, you can lay your ear on your patient's chest and listen for a heartbeat, but usually this is unnecessary. You will know when death has occurred. Rigor mortis (a stiffening of the body) sets in a few hours after death, usually starting in the jaw. Covering your patient's face is unnecessary. The eyes may remain opened or partially opened, but there is no need to close them. If you have taken your patient's dentures out prior to death, the mortician will want them, and you can place them in a covered denture cup.

Hopefully, you have been prepared for your patient's death and have discussed with the physician steps to take when your patient has died. (This will vary depending on location and the cause of death, so try to discuss this beforehand and if possible.) If you are uncertain about the steps to take following your patient's death, telephone your funeral director. He will be familiar with the laws in your state and will inform the proper authorities. Coroners have to be notified in certain cases.

▶ WHEN DYING AT HOME IS IMPOSSIBLE

In some instances it may not be feasible to care for your dying patient at home. Certainly if the person is in pain, you will want to discuss this with your physician. It may be suggested that your patient be transferred to a hospital or a nursing home, where he can be kept comfortable by more sophisticated means than you are able to provide at home. A hospice is sometimes recommended for the terminally ill patient. Even though you may not have fulfilled your patient's wish to die at home, take heart in the fact that you have done your very best to care for your patient during his stay with you and your family.

If your patient is transferred to a hospital or nursing home during the dying process, the subject of whether or not cardiopulmonary resuscitation (CPR) is to be performed will probably be brought up. CPR is external massage to the heart and supplying a mechanical means of breathing after the heart and lung function has ceased. Voice your opinion regarding the use of CPR. In some facilities CPR is performed unless it is specifically written on the patient's chart that family members have requested that it not be performed. If you are uncertain about these measures, discuss them with your physician.

▶ DEALING WITH GRIEF

You and your family will go through a period of grief or mourning after the death of your loved one. How you deal with grief is an individual matter. In some instances, especially if you knew your patient was dying, grief may have actually started before the patient died. The following is an example of how both a grieving patient and a caregiver dealt with grief.

Mr. J. is 79 years old and has suffered with crippling arthritis and heart disease for the past ten years. He is only able to walk 20 feet with his walker without becoming short of breath, and every movement is painful to his joints. For the past ten years, his wife had been caring for him in their own home. But suddenly, Mrs. J. became very ill and died. Mr. J. came to live with his daughter and son-in-law.

For Mr. J., this was the most emotionally traumatic time of his life. Not only did he have to cope with living in a new environment, but he was grieving the death of his wife. Consider, too, Mr. J.'s daughter who was also grieving the death of a loved one, plus having Mr. J. to care for. She did not know how to cope with her father's grief. When he first came, he spoke very little and only picked at his food.

At the loss of a loved one, the first response is numbness. The grieving person is unable to accept the fact that a loved one has actually died. Shock sets in, followed by the eventual reality that the loved one is really gone.

Mr. J. was still in shock. However, little by little, he became able to talk about his wife and his own loss. It helped both him and his daughter that they were together during this time and could share their grief.

The person suffering through grief may show great distress and become angry—even at you and your family. The grieving person may be irritable and nervous and will feel empty, hopeless, and desolate. Physically, the grieving person may have a loss of appetite, shortness of breath, insomnia, digestive problems or many other complaints. This stage of grief, however, begins to lessen in a month or two.

To overcome his grief, Mr. J. had to be able to express it. Crying is normal, and Mr. J.'s family needed to be sympathetic. Too often, the grieving widow or widower hears, "You must be brave now," from well-meaning friends. These words only help to suppress grieving. The grieving person feels he cannot cry or express grief since doing this would prove he is not brave.

Months after his wife's death, Mr. J. often made comments such as, "It should have been me. I should have been the one to die." After a time, Mr. J.'s daughter realized her father felt guilty about the fact that he was still alive while his wife, who had spent the last ten years of her life completely devoted to his care, was dead. The daughter's reply was to give him a hug, and say, "Dad, you were always wonderful to Mother. She used to tell us what a good husband you were. She didn't mind caring for you when you were sick because she loved you and she knew you loved her." Comments such as these helped Mr. J. through his grief and feelings of guilt.

While being understanding and tolerant of her father, Mr. J.'s daughter also helped by getting him involved again in normal patterns of living. Old friends began to visit and Mr. J. developed a friendship with another widower who lived on the next block. Their friendship deepened because they were both widowers and could discuss their problems. Visits from his pastor also helped.

Mr. J.'s daughter went through her own stages of grief over the death of her mother. Sometimes she cried with her father, and sometimes she cried alone. She found comfort in the fact that she had taken her father into her home to live, yet even though she had her father to care for, she became involved again with her normal patterns of living.

You have probably heard accounts of the grieving widow who still sets a plate at the table for her husband who died ten years ago. Such grieving is prolonged and abnormal. Within six months to a year the grieving period should largely be over. Any grief that seems to be prolonged should be reported to the physician to determine if a mental health program is needed.

If your loved one has just died, you will feel some of the emotions that Mr. J. and his daughter felt. Sometimes you will cry. There is an emptiness in your life. Seek the comfort of your family, friends, and clergyman during this time. If you think your grief has gone on for too long, ask for mental health counseling.

Thinking of your patient during the final stages of death may be painful. Instead, recall the good days. Remember that day you baked the patient's favorite dessert or the times you spent in his room talking and playing cards. Most importantly, seek consolation and take pride in the fact that your patient spent weeks, months, or even years living with you and your family in comfort, surrounded by love.

CHAPTER 14

SUMMARY: STRIVING FOR WELLNESS

You now have a basic background to administer good home care to your patient. In some instances you may be able to recognize signs and symptoms of illness before they become acute. You can save your patient pain and suffering, not to mention labor and stress on your part, by preventing problems common to the ill from occurring. To keep your patient as well and fit as possible, prevention, as always, is the best cure. Some general principles of wellness for you, your patient, and your family should always be applied.

1. Be consistent in your routine and care.
2. Keep regular doctor's appointments.
3. Keep regular dental appointments.
4. Have vaccines, such as influenza and pneumonia vaccines, administered if your physician suggests them.
5. Take medications as ordered.
6. Practice cleanliness in your home.
7. Practice cleanliness of yourself and your patient and wash hands frequently.

8. Eat a balanced diet.
9. If you smoke, quit.
10. Use alcohol in moderation.
11. Take off excess weight.
12. Safeguard your home according to your patient's needs.
13. Practice rules of safety while lifting, turning, and caring for your patient.
14. And specifically to the caring person and family who have offered your home to an ill person: Take good care of your own health. You are all very special.

APPENDIX A

LIQUIDS

3 teaspoons (tsp.) = 1 tablespoon (tbsp.)
2 tablespoons = 1 ounce (oz.)
8 ounces = 1 cup (c.)
4 cups = 1 quart (qt.)

U.S.	METRIC EQUIVALENT
1 teaspoon	5 cubic centimeters (cc)
2 tablespoons	30 cc
1 quart	1 liter (l) approx.

LENGTH

0.3937 inches (in.)	1 centimeter (cm)
39.37 inches	1 meter

APPENDIX B

▶ **HOME MEDICAL SUPPLY CATALOGS**

BRUCE MEDICAL SUPPLY
Dept. CFIH
411 Waverly Oaks Road
Waltham, MA 02154
1-800-225-8446
   Bathroom and Bedroom Supplies, Adaptive Tools for the Handicapped, Diabetic, Incontinence, Ostomy and Tracheostomy Needs. Free Catalog.

Comfortably Yours®
. . . Makes Living Easier™
61 West Hunter Avenue
Maywood, NJ 07607

SEARS Specialog HOME HEALTH CARE PRODUCTS
   This catalog is available at any local Sears store or write to:

SEARS, ROEBUCK AND CO.
925 S. Homan Avenue
Chicago, IL 60607

APPENDIX C

▶ **HEALTH INFORMATION CENTERS**

Alzheimer's Disease and Related Disorders Association
(800)621-0379
(800)572-6037 in IL only

American Diabetes Association
(800)227-6776
(212)683-7444 in NY

American Kidney Fund
(800)638-8299
(800)492-8361 in MD only

Arthritis Information Clearinghouse
P. O. Box 9782
Arlington, VA 22209
(703)558-8250

Cancer Information Service
(800)4-CANCER
(800)638-6070 in AK only
(800)636-5700 in DC area only
(808)524-1234 in Oahu, HI (Neighbor Islands call collect)

Epilepsy Information Line
(800)426-0660
(206)323-8174 in WA only

Hearing Helpline
(800)424-8576
(202)638-7577 in DC area only

Heartline
(800)241-6993
(404)523-0826 in GA only

National Association for Hearing and Speech Action Line
(800)638-8255
(301)897-8682 in HI, AK, and MD only (call collect)

National Hearing Aid Helpline
(800)521-5247
(313)478-2610 in MI only

National Institute of Mental Health
(301)443-4513

National Library Service for the Blind and Physically
    Handicapped
Library of Congress
Washington, DC 20542
(800)424-9100

National Second Surgical Opinion Program Hotline
(800)638-6833
(800)492-6603 in MD only

Parkinson's Education Program
(800)344-7872
(714)640-0218 in CA

APPENDIX D

SUGGESTED READING FOR PATIENTS AND CAREGIVERS

Books

The 36-Hour Day by Nancy L. Mace and Peter V. Rabins, Copyright 1981 by The Johns Hopkins University Press, Baltimore, MD 21218

Pamphlets

Alberto Culver Company furnishes information and recipes using Mrs. Dash. Write to:

Alberto Culver Company
2525 Armitage Avenue
Melrose Park, IL 60160

American Heart Association:

The American Heart Association Diet, An Eating Plan for Healthy Americans. 1985

Cholesterol and Your Heart. 1984

Sex and Heart Disease. 1983

Facts about Strokes

Salt, Sodium and Blood Pressure, Piecing Together the Puzzle. Chicago Heart Association, 1979

Heart Attack. 1975

Contact the local association for information and other pamphlets.

American Lung Association:

AROUND THE CLOCK WITH COPD. Booklet gives many helpful hints on how to live and cope with chronic obstructive pulmonary disease. For COPD patients. Assembled from actual daily practice by a support group for pulmonary patients. 32 pages, 1984.

CHRONIC BRONCHITIS FACTS and *EMPHYSEMA FACTS.* Leaflets explain symptoms, treatment, more. For the public and patients. 6 pages, 1986.

HELP YOURSELF TO BETTER BREATHING. Illustrated 28-page booklet that shows COPD patients and their families how to live more comfortably with the disease. Helps patients learn facts and deal with feelings, resources, and responsibilities. 1983.

All material copyright the American Lung Association—The Christmas Seal People®. Contact the local American Lung Association (listed in the white pages of the telephone directory) for information and other materials on lung diseases and their related causes.

BIBLIOGRAPHY

▶ BOOKS

Brunner, Lillian Sholtis, and Doris Smith Suddarth. *Textbook of Medical-Surgical Nursing.* 5th ed. Philadelphia: J. B. Lippincott, 1984.

Burnside, Irene Mortenson. *Psychosocial Nursing Care of the Aged.* 2d ed. New York: McGraw-Hill, 1980.

Butler, Robert N., and Myrna I. Lewis. *Aging and Mental Health.* 2d ed. St. Louis: The C. V. Mosby Company, 1977.

Hogstel, Mildred O., ed. *Nursing Care of the Older Adult.* New York: John Wiley & Sons, 1981.

Kohut, Sylvester, Jr., Jeraldine J. Kohut, and Joseph J. Fleishman. *Reality Orientation for the Elderly.* 2d ed. Oradel, New Jersey: Medical Economics Company Inc., 1983.

Kübler-Ross, Elizabeth. *On Death and Dying.* New York: Macmillan, 1969.

Mace, Nancy L., and Peter V. Rabins. *The 36-Hour Day.* Baltimore: The Johns Hopkins University Press, 1981.

Rambo, Beverly J., and Lucile A. Wood. *Nursing Skills for Clinical Practice.* 3d ed. Philadelphia: W. B. Saunders, 1982.

Springhouse Corporation. *Signs & Symptoms.* Nurse's Reference Library. Springhouse, Pa., 1986.

Steffl, Bernita M., ed. *Handbook of Gerontological Nursing.* New York: Van Nostrand Reinhold, 1984.

▶ BOOKLETS AND PAMPHLETS

About Alzheimer's Disease. The Pennsylvania Department of Aging. Channing L. Bete Co., Inc., South Deerfield, MA, 1985.

Alpert, Joseph S., and J. Dennis Mull. *Guide To Anticoagulant Therapy, Counseling and Follow-up.* E. I. DuPont de Nemours & Co. (Inc.), Wilmington, DE, 1984.

Bell, Martha Fenchak, and Charles C. Bell. *Aging and Senile Dementia.* Produced by Chronic Organic Brain Syndrome Society. Pennsylvania Department of Aging. No copyright.

Cholesterol and Your Heart. American Heart Association, 1984.

Emphysema. American Lung Association, 1984.

The Eye and Your Vision. NAVH Ophthalmological Advisory Board, Arthur H. Keeney, Chairman. National Association for Visually Handicapped, New York, 1978.

Nutrition an Ally in Cancer Therapy. Ross Laboratories, Columbus, OH, 1985.

Problems of the Partially Seeing. National Association for Visually Handicapped, New York, 1976.

Taking Care of Your Elderly Relatives. Channing L. Bete Co., Inc., South Deerfield, MA, 1983.

CREDIT
NOTES

1. Carnation Instant Breakfast is a product of the Carnation Company, Los Angeles, CA 90036.
2. Ensure® Liquid Nutrition is a product of Ross Laboratories, A Division of Abbott Laboratories, Columbus, OH 43216.
3. Mrs. Dash® is a registered trademark of the Alberto Culver Company, Melrose Park, IL 60160.
4. Fleet® Brand Ready to Use Disposable Enema and Fleet® Brand Ready to Use Mineral Oil Enema are registered copyrights of the C. B. Fleet Company, Inc., P. O. Box 11349, Lynchburg, VA 24506. Information regarding the use and administration of the Fleet® Enema is approved by the C. B. Fleet Company, Inc.
5. Pepto-Bismol® is a product of Norwich Eaton Pharmaceuticals, Inc., Distributed by Procter & Gamble, Cincinnati, OH 45202.
6. Coumadin® is a registered trademark of E. I. duPont de Nemours & Co. (Inc.), Wilmington, DE 19898.
7. The National Association for Visually Handicapped (NAVH) is a nonprofit voluntary health agency. NAVH has helped supply information and has approved the text regarding low vision problems and visual aids.

INDEX